AIDS:

From Fear To Hope

**Channeled Teachings
Offering
Insight and Inspiration**

SPIRIT SPEAKS

Layout, Design, and Graphics by:

On Line Graphics, Inc., Miami, Florida

Cover Design and Illustration by: **Sushila Jean Oliphant**

Rainbow Concept by: **Joan W. Segal**

First Printing

ISBN: 0-934619-02-6

Dedication

To all the divinely human beings
who are affected by
the phenomenon called AIDS.

"In your hand you hold some possible answers to your questions about AIDS. It is so important for you to read this material, because nowhere else is anyone approaching it from so many perspectives.

We are Spirit Teachers working with channels and others for the comfort and care of the Planet Earth; helping to cure the sadness, the fear, the pain and the unrest.

Remember to love yourselves. Remember to love each other. And keep yourself going ever strongly forward."

–The Spirit Teachers

Acknowledgment

Special thanks from **"Spirit Speaks Publications"** *to:*

Steve Bolme, Nancy Elkins, Mercy Kieffer, Gary Lund, Sharon MacDonald, Glenn Nickell, Paula Nowels, Laura Spickler, Randy Spickler, Karla Spitzer and **Marty Segal.** Their dedicated hours of labor and enthusiasm for this project helped bring the original workbook, **"AIDS: Spirits Share Understanding and Hope from the 'other' Side"** to life as this book which you now hold in your hands.

Special thanks from **David Hecht:**

For my best friend, **Dan Bradley,** courageously living with AIDS–for being part of my spiritual awakening, my transformation and for allowing me to open my heart to life and for giving me the gift of love.

Contents

ix

x

Author's Preface

Thank you for opening this book. Not too many years ago I would not have had the courage to consider reading a book of this nature unless it was either scientifically backed or authored by someone with alphabet soup initials after their name. Unwilling to accept things on faith or according to my feelings, I demanded proof before I could believe anything.

This constant need for validity came from a very basic and deep belief that I was alone in a hostile Universe. Scared of life, unwilling to face my deepest feelings and fears, I was terrified of the "black hole" of death. I prided myself on being a practicing agnostic, denying the existence of God. Always one to hedge my bets, I was unwilling to be a full-fledged atheist, just in case I was wrong.

In March, 1982, I attended a "channeled" lecture and was introduced to an incredibly loving and wise teacher, a Spirit being named Dr. Peebles. He spoke on families, children, and the choices we make before coming into physical life. When the lecture was finished, I was transformed. The information shared that evening touched me, moved me, and helped me peek at my inner feelings and beliefs for the first time. Most importantly, I had discovered there was a distinct possibility that I was not alone, but part of a loving, joyful, eternal, perfect God. What an incredible surprise! Wanting to know more, I read as much channeled material as I could locate (no easy task in 1982). Eventually I enrolled in a mediumship class and discovered

1

that channeling, sometimes regarded as a rather strange practice, was not strange at all, but a natural communication ability that everyone has and can develop at will.

The position shift which I experienced is being duplicated by millions of so-called "normal" people who are discovering there is something beyond the physical—intelligence and communication from life forms in other dimensions. They welcome this communication as a gift of insight and assistance as they face the challenges of physical life.

The information in this book is an offering of insight, a sharing of comfort, hope, and love. No strings, no hidden catches. My publishing associates and I come from mainstream America. We all were non-believers in this "spirit speaking" business until we were exposed to it and had the opportunity to incorporate the information and techniques into our daily lives. If you can, for just a moment, set aside any pre-conceived notions about channeled information, and look at the material on these pages. Allow the words to speak to you. Most likely you will find a pearl of wisdom that touches your heart because it speaks a truth for you. And then you'll find another one, and another. Soon, like a treasure hunt, you'll have a string of pearls which will bring you greater understanding about yourself, about love, about life, about AIDS.

And, if you still feel skeptical, that's all right. You need to be comfortable with whatever you believe. Former skeptics all, we understand your point of view. However, if you find a slight crack appearing in that skepticism, we encourage you to really *read* this book, and then other materials which will come your way. We encourage you to find out more about yourself, why you're here, where you're from, and why you have made certain choices about your life experiences.

As AIDS moves across our planet, many people are filled with despair by the bleak points of view offered by theologians, physicians, and scientists. Their limited viewpoints, shouting to the public through the media, are creating tremendous anxiety, fear, uncertainty, and confusion. To serve the need for a *broader perspective* about AIDS, my associates and I, in a collective effort, compiled,

2

transcribed, and edited over 60 hours of channeled teachings to create this book.

Our original plan was to assemble material about AIDS, and as we compiled the material, it became clear that it was impossible to separate this illness from all other aspects of life. Therefore, we have included background information about the purpose of living as a human being on the planet Earth, the choices we make before incarnating, and how every event in our lives is interconnected with every other event and every other living being. Understanding these choices and connections with all life can be soothing and helpful in understanding not only AIDS, but all life experiences.

We do not present this material in a proselytizing "we have all the answers" spirit. We simply offer you loving, clear, and helpful information from our Spirit associates.

You may not be aware of exactly what the term "channeling" means and how it was used to create this book. Channeling, as a communication process, is an ancient one, newly revived. It is a viable method that brings helpful information forth from the collective consciousness. This information has *always* been available to mankind, but, until recently, it only has been utilized by those aware of it and able to receive it without apprehension.

For many years, scientists have recognized that energy is the basis for all life in the Universe. This energy has been identified as a mass of consciousness containing all knowledge and all wisdom of this Earth and, in fact, of the entire Universe. Plato, Jung, Einstein, and others have described the collective consciousness as an endless pool of energy and knowledge. You might liken it to a Universal television station, endlessly broadcasting. Just as we can tune our television channels to programs of interest, we can also tune in to conscious intelligence existing in a reality located beyond our usual means of communication.

Prophets in Biblical times openly acknowledged their communication and inspiration as being received from those of the Angelic realms. For the past hundred years, those who brought forward information from any non-physical dimension were called trance mediums, mystics, or sensitives. Today we call them channels, a term used to describe how they channel information from one dimension to another. Channels are trained to step aside from their normal state of consciousness, moving into what scientists refer to as an "altered state." While in this altered state, they allow, by *agreement* and in *complete cooperation,* spirit energies (we call them Spirit Teachers) to speak through them for brief periods of time.

More and more people are becoming aware of channeling as a source of increased knowledge, and are anxious to read the teachings brought forth via this process. The Edgar Cayce books, still popular 30 years after his death, attest to the deep-seated interest millions have regarding guidance and wisdom from the spirit dimension. A survey in early 1987 reported that at least 95 million Americans believed they had lived before. In Shirley MacLaine's TV movie "Out On A Limb" (viewed by 35 million Americans), she utilized channeled information as a gentle and comfortable guide for starting on her personal, internal quest of increased awareness.

Spirit Teachers who speak via the channeling process are compassionate beings, eager to help us more fully understand our relationship to daily trials and tribulations. Most Spirit Teachers have occupied physical bodies themselves and are acutely aware of the frustrations and fears we experience. They desire to communicate with us because they wish to assist us in remembering more about *who we are* and *why we have chosen* to experience physical life. Because they are not (at the moment) in physical form, they see life on the planet Earth from a broader perspective than we do as we struggle with the complexities of daily living. They desire to offer a helping hand to better prepare us for continual social, economic, physical, and environmental changes. Their alternative points of view are easy to read and frequently contain doses of humor and a familiarity about life which give us greater *understanding* renewed *hope* and increased *comfort* about our various roles in the human experience.

There are hundreds and thousands of different groups of Spirit Teachers devoting their energy and love toward the upliftment of all humanity and the healing of the planet Earth. However, for purposes of clear communication, only one Spirit Teacher represents each

4

group (which is why they refer to themselves as "we").

The most important message that all Spirit Teachers have for us is that we have *chosen* to be physical human beings. They teach that in life, there are *no victims. There are only creators.* They stress that we have chosen to be physical for the express purpose of gaining *greater understanding* of all aspects of life.

Basically, we set up our lives with specific experiences in mind. It's much like making plans for a trip to summer camp. First you evaluate available information (brochures) to determine which camp suits your desires most completely. Perhaps you decide to travel to a foreign country to experience the adventure of not being able to communicate with others until a new language is learned from scratch. When the appointed time arrives, you take a little trip to your destination. At first it is a little awkward communicating, but with assistance from the counselors and other campers, you catch on. Now, sometimes, the best laid plans. . . you know how that goes. You may experience the measles, and spend your entire vacation learning French by reading novels in the infirmary. But, you do get your experience, although it may not be *exactly* as you had planned. When camp is over, everybody hugs and cries and promises to write and off you go, back home again. You share photographs and experiences with your family, and before you know it, you're making plans to attend another camp to experience a different type of adventure.

Life is like this. . . at least mostly. There are a few differences. You make your plans depending on what you want to experience. You take a little trip (being born), and suddenly find yourself in a foreign country, slightly paralyzed, unable to speak the language, and with amnesia. So, you take a few years to learn language, communication and motor skills, and with your Spirit Guides and physical parents at your side, you pursue chosen experiences. If you travel far afield from your chosen experiences, those around you help you move back onto your chosen path. When it's all over, you go home by experiencing the transition called "death" and are born again on the spirit side. You share experiences with your spirit family and friends, and before too long, you're making plans to do it all again.

Although this explanation is a bit simplistic, it does present the basic concept of *free will and choice* which is highly individual according to the experiential needs of each individual.

All Spirit Teachers have experienced widely different life situations, chosen for the learning involved. This great variety in experience creates multiple points of view. Therefore, some of their statements, on the surface, may appear to be contradictory. Consider this: if you asked eleven people to study a rose, then describe it, you would receive eleven different responses. One person would comment on the thorns, another on the stem, yet another on the aroma. All would see aspects of the whole flower from different perspectives. When you put these aspects together, they complement each other rather than contradict. So, when you find passages in this book which seem to be contradictory, remember the rose. Then listen to that still, small voice within your heart to find the truths which are perfect for your unique and special level of understanding.

In the words of one of our Spirit contributors, Dong How Li, "Please remember, take what resonates with you, what assists, what nourishes, what feeds you; above all, what inspires you to do what you have come to do. The rest, please leave by the wayside."

All involved in the creation of this book send you light and love and encouragement.

Molli Nickell,
Editor-in-Chief, **Spirit Speaks Publications**
Los Angeles, California
July, 1987

Publisher's Introduction

"We are embarked upon a New Age of insight, awareness, co-operation and growth. We have great dreams, and the opportunity to make them come true."

–The Motto of New Age Publishing Co.

Today, book stores are filled with New Age works on many diverse subjects. New Age music occupies large sections in our record stores and wins Grammy awards. We are attending lectures and workshops on personal growth and elevation of consciousness in increasing numbers. Traditional print media and network television present articles, features and prime time shows on many philosophical and psychological matters. Holistic health, nutrition and exercise are increasingly pursued and endorsed by the medical profession. Scientists acknowledge the connection between quantum physics and the metaphysical workings of the Universe. Documented reports of psychic phenomena abound.

One senses a quickening of the collective energy, as the quest for personal growth and fulfillment is accelerating. There is growing inquiry into basic issues of life and into the meaning of existence. It is becoming increasingly apparent that our focus is changing.

Many of us have tired of playing the game of seeking our answers in the exterior world of recreational diversions and illusive promises of lasting happiness. The new car, new job or new relationship still doesn't give us that sense of peace, contentment and real meaning that we intuitively seek.

This sometimes desperate search to find happiness "out there" in the material world is coming to the realization that the most important answers lie within. Perhaps it is a sense of peril, not only for themselves but for the planet, that has propelled so many into seeking new answers to old questions, new solutions for personal problems and new understandings of themselves. Our circular journey seeking truth seems to be headed back home.

And yet, amidst this encouraging background of expanded consciousness and awareness, there rises the dark and foreboding spectrum of AIDS. It has seemingly paralyzed us with anxiety. All forms of media recount its daily spread, the effect being a corresponding increase in the level of fear and helplessness permeating society. A random sampling of its growing impact on our everyday lives can be felt by looking at the main topics of discussion in daily newspapers, leading magazines, radio talk shows, television forums and wire service news. There is daily speculation about the problem without any suggested effective solutions.

One must travel back to the Middle Ages and the Black Plague which swept the Continent to experience a similar climate. The paradox is that our world is experiencing so much illumination in its search for truth, yet it is now faced with this challenge of apparent darkness.

But what is darkness but the absence of light? The projection of a beam of light automatically dispels the dark. It is obvious that we desperately need a new and enlightened perspective on this subject if real healing is to occur and practical solutions are to be forthcoming. What are the lessons to be learned from the AIDS problem? Why has it manifested at this time? Is there a solution? What should we do?

We must expand our viewpoint beyond traditional medical and religious explanations. They are only adding to the fear and negativity as the problem persists and grows. We need an overview of the entire situation that presents an expanded viewpoint of wisdom and understanding. This can only come from sources of information beyond our limited three-dimensional focus. Fortunately, such higher wisdom is now available through the communication process called "channeling," explained in the Author's Preface and in Part II.

The Spirit Teachers are our friends. They want to help us.We receive the benefit of their wisdom on the subjects which they address, like a panel of experts who present a personal symposium of knowledge for our assistance.

This book examines the AIDS phenomena in particular, from the vantage point of life in general. It reflects the delicate inter-relationships between all of us as we try to understand the meaning of our lives and find ways to enhance our experience of living. It suggests that there is a connection between all the major events of our lives—a master plan for our personal evolution based upon experience and understanding. In this overview, we are all striving for the same goals and traveling in the same direction, even though our paths may differ.

The series of meaningful coincidences that resulted in the production of this book are a case in point for the linkage we all share as human beings. **New Age Publishing Co.** was formed in 1985 and published my book entitled **"THE GURU IS YOU: How to Play, and Win, the Game of Life"** in 1986. The book was a personal and pragmatic sharing of ways to increase one's enjoyment of life through positive inner direction. It contained first-hand experiences of channeling.

In the same year, a group of people in California, headed by Molli Nickell, decided to present channeled material in a monthly magazine format called **"Spirit Speaks."** Their stated purpose was "to share guidance and wisdom from the loving beings of the Spirit Plane." Her group works closely with numerous contributing channels, receiving their taped or written sharings on assigned topics. Since the information is spoken to be heard, it requires editing for the speech patterns of distant or foreign incarnations, and is then reviewed, and presented in separate issues that address a particular monthly topic. In the course of their work, Molli's group received quite a bit of material from the channels concerning AIDS, who felt it important that this information be presented to the public. It was compiled and presented in a ring-binder book format in 1986 under the title **"AIDS: Spirits Share Understanding and Hope from the 'Other' Side."**

I became a subscriber to **"Spirit Speaks"** due to my interest in channeling, and the quality of the material offered. Molli became aware of my company through my book, and we exchanged thoughts about the publication of an edited, revised and updated version of the AIDS book as a quality paperback with worldwide distribution.

At the same time, David Hecht, a successful Miami businessman and a leading member of the San Francisco gay community, had recently become interested in consciousness growth, and had also read my book. We discussed it and I brought Molli's AIDS book to his attention. He was enthused about its value as an inspiring and helpful work, of special interest to the gay community. He was interested in collaborating with my company in the new AIDS book project.

The three of us met, discussed the project in greater detail, and resolved to proceed. **New Age Publishing Co.** purchased from **"Spirit Speaks"** the worldwide rights to their original book, and formed a business association with David for publication of the new work. The existing book was extensively edited, reworked, and revised. Pertinent material from prior issues of **"Spirit Speaks"** magazine, was adapted. New channeled material, never before published, was received from the contributing channels and incorporated in the book. Extensive design, graphics, artwork and layout were completed, all resulting in the finished work which you see before you.

A final synchronous event was the cover design. It was important to use the color spectrum for the cover, to signify the hopeful emergence of this subject from darkness to light. Channelings received after that decision had identical suggestions and urged us to emphasize color:

"The more colorful you can get the cover, the better—something that draws people's eye to it–but with joy in it. And upbeat—it must be upbeat. It must stress the possibility and hope behind it."

10

A triad of these meaningful coincidences was completed when David pointed out that the official flag of the gay community is, in fact, the rainbow.

So I bid you welcome, and hope that you find much food for thought that will be of assistance in nourishing you as you journey down life's highway. Any portion of the material is perfect if it resonates within you. May your outlook be transformed "from fear to hope." My colleagues and I wish you all the very best in your travels.

Martin E. Segal, President
New Age Publishing Co.
Miami, Florida
July, 1987

Introducing The Spirit Teachers
And
Their Channels

"The Spirit Teachers want to help us...We receive the benefit of their wisdom on the subjects they address, like a panel of experts who present a personal symposium of knowledge for our assistance."

–Publisher's Introduction

1. **Enid**—last lived in the physical plane in the 1840's in Ireland, at which time she awakened to higher consciousness. She speaks in an earthy, warm manner with an Irish brogue. She is channeled by Iris Belhayes, author of "Spirit Guides," who resides in Los Angeles, California.

2. **Dr. Peebles**—was last incarnated in Scotland in the 1800's, and, after years of medical practice in England, came to the United States to research the philosophic basis of illness and accident. He is channeled by Reverend William Rainen, who resides in Tempe, Arizona.

3. **Dong How Li**—is a spiritual counselor and philosopher who was last incarnated as a Tibetan monk in the Nepalese Himalayas in 600 B.C. He is channeled by Reverend Allen Page, who resides in Glendale, California.

4. **Kyros**—is a spirit being who has not previously chosen to express in a physical existence. His channel is Sandra J. Radhoff, a co-founder of the "Universalia" channeling study group in Colorado. She resides in Lakewood, Colorado.

5. **Master Adalfo**—last lived as an artist in renaissance Italy. His philosophy comes from influence of prior lifetimes spent as a priest and scientist on the continent of Atlantis. He is channeled by Reverend Carol Simpson, who resides in Northridge, California.

6. **Soli**—is an off-planet being from the Pleiades. He is channeled by Reverend Neville Rowe, a graduate electrical engineer born in New Zealand, who now resides in West Hollywood, California.

7. **Taulmus**—is a being from the Pleiades star system on a voyage from his home planet, to share his expanded viewpoint and loving concern with mankind. He is channeled by Salli Lou West, who resides in Santa Fe, New Mexico.

8. **Ting-Lao**—was last incarnated 2,000 years ago and expresses his personality as an oriental philosopher and teacher. He is channeled by Reverend Kris Topaz who holds college degrees in Human Development. She resides in Pasadena, California.

9. **Zoosh**—is a non-physical, energy personality being from Alpha Centauri, the nearest star to our sun. He is channeled by Robert Shapiro, who also channels a spirit being named **Jesus of the Light**, who is a part of the Christ consciousness. Robert resides in Durango, Colorado, and is the author of "Allies," a book about off-planet beings.

I

How The Universe Really Works

"You daily create your reality. What you think, what comes forward within your subconscious mind constantly, is what you'll see around you. If you think you are poor, then you'll be poor. If you think you're unloved and unlovely, then you will have no one around you. You receive back exactly what you put out. Whatever you believe, you will have, regardless of what it is.

It is important that you recognize that there is no experience that comes into your life that is below your dignity, or below your exploration. It is for you to acknowledge that no matter what comes into your life, it is little more than an educational experience and each and every experience is an opportunity for you to re-evaluate your total enlightenment."

1

We Are Spirit

Soli

You are not your physical bodies. You are not your emotions. You are not your intellects. You are your Higher Selves. You are Spirit. You are a Spirit experiencing the physical dimension through the vehicle of a physical body. It is as though you were planning to travel to San Francisco, and needed to rent a vehicle in which to go there. You find one, rent it and make that trip. When you come back from that journey, you return the vehicle to the rental agency. If you decide on another trip, you again go through that same process: you choose a destination and the vehicle in which to travel in. There are infinite destinations, as well as infinite vehicles.

It is in much the same way that one arrives on the Earth plane. Obviously, it is not quite as simple as this; however, this gives you a general idea of incarnation. You choose your physical vehicle, you use it for the extent of this life and then you leave it behind when you go. You also choose a particular place, time and family, for a particular experience needed by your Higher Self in order to evolve. This is not your only existence. There have been countless lives, because, as a living Spirit, your Higher Self is experiencing through you. It is the subconscious mind and its belief systems that try to tell you that you are the isolated individual that you think you are, that what is all around you is all that is, and that what you have within your physical body is all there is of you.

17

This is an illusion, my friends. This is what the spiritual teachers refer to as "Maya," or cosmic illusion. Your reality is that of an *unlimited, infinite, and indestructible Spirit with perpetual existence.*

Zoosh

How many times have you been told that we are all one Spirit, that we are all one consciousness, that we are all one being? Understand that we are, indeed, all one. There is no separation whatsoever. There is only an illusion of separation. To understand this better, understand that the cells in your finger do not have any particular understanding that they are cells within a finger operating a muscle, tissue, bone or whatever. They do not have the consciousness to know that they are cells within a finger and yet your finger functions as it is a part of your hand, as it is a part of your arm, as it is a part of your body. And yet, would you say that your finger is a separate entity unto itself, that each cell is a separate entity? In one manner of looking at it, you might say that each cell is, indeed, separate. And yet, together they function very nicely as a finger, as a hand, and as a body, and so on.

So, in this sense, you can truly understand that each of you is a cell in the "All That Is." In your body, there are millions and millions of cells just as there are millions and millions of souls and light bodies around the Universe. They are all cells, in that sense, within a massive body of consciousness.

2

Satisfying Your Need For Experience

Dr. Peebles

Recognize always, my friends, that life is a delightful opportunity to experience growth and change that leads you always to the higher levels of fulfillment. Visualize, my friends, that you, while on the Spirit side of life, chose exactly who and what you are today. You chose the experiences, the environments, the circumstances, the collective consciousness of the time that would give you the opportunity to participate in the fulfillment of the karmic destiny of the planet Earth through its collective consciousness and also to attain the fulfillment of your soul. Recognize that this is but a stepping-stone to a higher and more complete enlightenment, and if you attain fulfillment in this life, it is for you to embrace the light of your soul, to embrace all that you have ever been, all that you are, and all that you will ever become, once more.

It is important that you recognize that there is no experience that comes into your life that is below your dignity, or below your exploration. It is for you to acknowledge that *no matter what* comes into your life, it is little more than an educational experience and each and every experience is an *opportunity* for you to re-evaluate your total enlightenment.

Be aware, my friends, that whatever experience comes into your life, it is not for your own growth alone. Anything or anyone who is affected by an experience related to you is ultimately part of the balancing system. You must, then, always be willing to embrace the input of vibrations, thoughts and ideas of all the life forms on the planet Earth. For then, all will be able to grow. Recognize, then, that there are only valid questions, although there is a tendency to embrace invalid answers. Answers are often created out of logic and have little, if anything, to do with the answers already in motion on the soul and Spirit level.

Soli

There really is no purpose to life apart from experiencing it. There is no purpose to anything. There is no purpose to suffering or happiness except to experience it. It just is. But there is cause and effect. If you have a certain belief system or do a certain act, then there is an effect from that. There is no purpose within the act or the effect, except to give you the experience of that act, by showing you what the act is, and for you to experience the power of your own creativity through thought within the physical dimension. Therefore, nothing is more important than anything else. Everything is infinite. There is no time and space. If you don't do it in this lifetime, you will do it in the next.

It is not important in one sense. However, in the sense of your subconscious mind, it becomes important in your daily lives. In the short, narrow view of the physical plane, these things become important, but on a higher level, in the wider perspective of the spiritual, nothing is more important than anything else. All are equal.

There is only one belief to hold on to, only one belief that you actually need in life and that is, *"I AM THAT I AM. I AM GOD. I AM EVERYTHING. I AM ALREADY PERFECTION."* Now, if you hold these thoughts constantly in your consciousness, all else falls into place automatically. You do not need to do anything else at all, for then you know your God-Self, and you allow that energy to come forward in life.

It is very simple. Simplicity is the key to evolution. Yet, of course, human beings want to complicate the simplest of things. This is what logic and intellect do. This is the role they play. If it is simple, it is obviously wrong. It is too easy. There must be a more complicated answer. It cannot possibly be so simple. Yet it is. It is letting go of concepts and belief systems. It is by going beyond the subconscious projections through meditation, and communicating directly with your Higher Self. Talk to your Higher Self. Feel the energy of your Higher Self. Know that this is truly you and it is God. Know that you and God are the *same* thing.

Those who choose to incarnate within the Earth plane do so because they want a very intense physical experience. They want to have that strong cut-off from the Spirit. However, in cutting off from the Spirit, people have forgotten their true spiritual origin. And this is what creates *dis-ease* on the Earth plane. For there is somewhere deep within you an understanding of your true origin. There arises a longing for that re-unification with the Spirit and God and with all life, of which you are an integral part. God expresses through you on the Earth plane.

Enid

Understand that life on this plane is lived on different levels. For example there is a higher part of you that is applauding your experience for your willingness to dig deep into the physical experience. And all beings who come here come for the expressed purpose of expanding their experience so that they will have a wonderful richness and expansion to fall back on when they go back to life as Spirits. With this fullness of experience, they are in a better position to be more helpful to others. There have been experiences in your own life, in the past, that have forever changed your view of yourself and your view of life. Well, that is what you take with you when you leave the body. You take all the richness of experience, all the greater depth of understanding. You see, you really can take it with you!

Also, understand that since you live a *snowflake* kind of existence, you are different and unique from any other, just as your fingerprints are different. It is a mark of your separateness and your ability to experience separation. However, all the "snowflakes" are created by

21

and fall from a common source. They are both separate and interconnected. On this level, all of life's experiences are later shared with all other beings in existence because we are all one, as related parts of this common source.

The only things that really truly happen, happen within the self, deep inside your heart. So, your experience, whether you realize it or not, (if you analyze it you'll know deep within your heart that it's true) will affect all other life. All other life will gain by the depth of your experience, although you may feel there is nothing wonderful about pain or devastation of the body or watching the body change before your eyes. I know how this feels, you see. I know how you feel in what you are experiencing.

Know that if this experience was not real to you, and if it wasn't felt with great depth, you would never gain what you wanted to gain from it. In order to experience this at all, you have been masterful in creating a state of reality for yourself in which it could happen.

We are experiencing the Earth dimension because there is no other place to find out the things that we can find out here.

There is no other place where you can step on a rusty nail.

There is no other place where you can see the sunset as you can see it here.

There is no other place where you can enjoy the feeling of water lapping upon your feet on the beach and feel the sand falling out from under your foot.

There is no other place where you can look into the truest eyes of your lover and bring the bodies together with such communion.

There is no other place that you can feel the pangs of loneliness and later come into your own and realize that you were never alone.

22

The great adventure, of course, is to come back to your own true self.

The great adventure, of course, is to do what you're doing now, rejoining your spirituality.

3

The Process Of Incarnation

Dr. Peebles

When you were on the Spirit side of life, your total consciousness, unrelated to your present personality, evaluated the circumstances and the events that have been an intricate part of your growth. Your soul determined that there were certain experiences, certain obligations, certain debts, certain gifts that you must experience and could experience. You looked down upon the Earth and you discovered the physical vehicles that would give you certain tendencies, that would put you into certain environments and cultures, that would allow you to have not only your individual experiences, but also your experiential events, so that you would enter life well-equipped to go about the business of balancing and of starting the ultimate release.

Now, to accomplish this, it is necessary to pass through what we call the *Valley of Forgetfulness*. This is a time when your total soul enters into a cleansing so that when you are born, as you develop, you will not over influence yourself. You also will not over influence the free will of others. You will be able to determine what is apropos for yourself according to that which is most in harmony with your soul's evolution.

Soli

The Higher Self chooses a path of growth on the Earth plane. In

24

order to do this, it has to funnel itself down. The high vibrational energy funnels down into a small, screwed-up ball, as it were, and finds itself locked up, once again, within the prison of a physical body. The Earth plane consists of the densest and lowest vibration of any within the Universe. This is a fact, not a judgment; it just is. So, through the Higher Self, you channel your energies down into this physical body through choice, and in doing so, you cut yourself off from your spiritual origin.

This move is the farthest from the understanding of your true spiritual nature, and of the understanding of God; however, you have chosen to have this experience. You begin to move further away from your spiritual origin as your subconscious mind becomes more and more programmed. As a child, you begin to remember less and less of your origin. It is absolute nonsense to say that a child is innocent because when the Spirit comes into the physical body, it remembers the previous life, or lives, and sometimes very strongly. The loss of the memory of those lives begins as the subconscious mind becomes more and more programmed, as if a veil of forgetfulness were drawn across it.

As you understand your previous incarnations, and analyze those experiences that you've had, you then decide on the experiences that you still require within the physical plane. You decide within the spiritual dimension, while working with your Guides and Teachers, on the parents that you will have, on the time and the place, the society, and the country in which you will live, with the full knowledge of all the probability patterns that you will be faced with throughout your life. Probabilities, my friends, not certainties, for you always have free will and choice in every action.

Your memory is your recording device. The subconscious mind is clear, clean, and new. It has not been used when you bring it into your physical body. From the moment you incarnate, that recording device begins to record all the signals from the five senses: taste, touch, sight, smell, sound, plus others. It also begins to record all the signals from the sixth sense as well, such as all those things that you are conscious of, that are recorded within the subconscious mind. You are conscious of them fleetingly and then you forget them, but they are

25

stored there and continue to act within your life for the rest of your life. You continue to be run by those programs within the subconscious.

All the belief systems of the society that you grew up in, the deep-seated religious beliefs that are part of that society, those things that you hear your parents and friends discussing when they do not think you are listening: these all become a part of your belief system, too, even if you do not know they are there. You know they are there later in life when you start to find reactions coming forward to actions that you are making. Then you begin to feel or discover that you have beliefs and thought forms that you never knew you had.

Where do they come from? They come from the time you incarnated. All those years as a child were when you were being indoctrinated. And that is what some would call "brain washing." Of course, it is all by your own choice for that belief system is what you knew you'd have. It is what you required. Those parents, those friends of parents, those teachers and the society you live in were what you required. The probability patterns upon the Earth plane, were needed by you for the experiences you require within your evolution for your personal growth.

You choose the genetic pattern of the body that you will inhabit. In some instances, you have modified or affected the body while it was still within the womb so that it will closely match your needs upon this planet. Therefore, those who are termed "handicapped" by society, by the masses, are only projections of society's subconscious minds. Society is making a judgment, looking through their limited minds and saying, "Look at that person; he is handicapped." This is nonsense. There is no such thing as a handicapped person. There is only experience. There is only growth. There is only evolution. There is always a choice.

Incarnation can begin any time between conception and approximately two months after birth. You chose the time of your incarnation just as you chose the time of your physical birth. Again, it is by your choice that you determine those aspects of the physical that you will be dealing with here on Earth. All this gives you the probability patterns that you need for your evolution. You know exactly the type of programming or teaching that you will receive from your parents. You know their friends and the type of society in which they live. You also have knowledge of the belief systems that you will grow up with because they are programmed within your own subconscious mind from the very moment that you incarnate, even before your actual birth.

4

Creating Your Own Reality–
The Power Of Thought

Soli

Having come to this Earth plane, you have chosen a particular physical body in order to perceive the world in a certain way. First the thought arises, then time, place and a physical body to carry out that thought. First comes the thought, then comes the reality. It is not the other way around as the masses have taught you. *Whatever you think, so you become.* Your individual thought creates your own environment within the mass environment. The reality of the mass environment, all that you see around you, is the consensus reality of all your brothers and sisters who have also incarnated here. Anyone who has ever had an interest in the Earth plane, or who has ever thought about the Earth plane, is helping to create the consensus reality, or mass consciousness, that you see around you in the world.

Your thoughts, my friends, are tools of power. Do you look in the mirror in the morning, when you wake, and say, "My goodness, I am getting old! My hair is turning gray; I have lines under my eyes; my body is falling apart." If you tell yourself this each day, then you are creating that reality for yourself, and you will age before your time. If, however, you repeat, "I see a radiant and beautiful being! I see a physical body that matches closely that perfection that I already am," then you are creating that reality, and you become radiant, beautiful and healthy.

Thoughts create your bodies. Thoughts create the cells. The cells in your bodies are being constantly changed. Moment to moment, you are never the same individual. Your body is not the same. Most believe their cells are going to deteriorate as time goes by, that their bodies have to age as time goes by. You are programmed, my friends, to believe that you are going down the hill past the age of 20. You are programmed to believe that after the age of 65, or even 55, you are not worthy anymore, that you are of no use to anyone, and you must retire.

Another example, if your mother used to tell you continuously that you will catch a cold if you get your feet wet in the rain, then, for the rest of your life you will definitely get a cold every time you get your feet wet in the rain! There is absolutely no reasoning behind this. You get your hands wet all the time, why should you get a cold only when your feet are wet? Yet, this is a very dearly held belief system and because this belief system is so strong, it has become the reality of a large number of people. Those are belief systems, my friends. To the extent that you believe in them, to that extent they become your reality.

What you see around you is your own projection of your subconscious mind. Those things that you deal with daily, such as your interactions with friends and acquaintances, all stem from subconscious projections and beliefs that you have.

Firstly, you must recognize that you have these beliefs and also recognize that the subconscious mind has this power, and that your body and its so-called illnesses or diseases are created by your subconscious projections which are brought forward by your belief systems in direct response.

Become conscious of those belief systems which are controlling your life. Become conscious of the thought forms that you repeat daily, for those thought forms create your reality, and they also create the negativity that you see around you. Become conscious of them and then change them. You can change them through meditation and specific affirmations; these are very important methods. However, you must also try to catch those negative thoughts that come forward in your day-to-day life, and turn them around. Tell yourself that you have no need to deal with them any longer.

My friends, why are you here? What are you doing upon this Earth plane? First and foremost, you decide to incarnate and, at that instant, to forget that you are already one with God, that you are already perfection, that you are already one with all life, that you are already *immortal, eternal, infinite and universal.*

You are on the path to the higher source. You will be remembering and reconnecting with the higher source, and in the process experiencing delightful and not-so-delightful aspects of the Earth plane along the way. As you learn to bring forward more of the Higher Self throughout your daily life, you will experience the physical dimension in its fullness. Allow that inner power, that brightness, that light, and that God force that you are to shine forward during your life, your day, so that the subconscious mind has less and less effect upon your life.

Do not fight the subconscious mind, as you do not fight yourself. The subconscious mind is your storehouse, your memory, your ego of this lifetime. It is necessary. *You are here to walk with it.* Once you have gone totally beyond the subconscious, when you have no more subconscious reaction within your life, then there's no longer any point to being upon the Earth plane. You will move on to the next dimension of experience.

And, so, my friends, you daily create your reality. What you think, what comes forward within your subconscious mind constantly, is what you'll see around you. If you think you are poor, then you'll be poor. If you think you're unloved and unlovely, then you will have no one around you. It is your fault, your belief. You receive back exactly what you put out. Whatever you believe, you will have, regardless of what it is. Why, then, not turn that thought around?

Give love. *Believe you are loved and you will be.* Believe and know and understand that you are one with the Universe and abundance is yours, and it will be. There is no limit, my friends; you can do anything. You can walk on water, you can swim in the Earth. You can do it! It is your belief that says you cannot or you can. That is *all* it is. Literally, without limitation, whatever you believe totally is your reality. Absolutely. That is why we say there is no one truth. As you change your beliefs, then your truth changes. If you would look

30

around you within society and judge others, what you are saying is, "That person's life does not match my belief system. They are wrong."

What do you do when you do that? You draw yourself into conflict with that vibration. If you feel that you are a victim of crime, or a criminal, it is because you have drawn an energy to you either through the fear that it would happen, or because you have some need in your life that you are not addressing and the only way that the Higher Self can get you to address that is to create within your life a situation that will force you to address it. So, the apparent individual who's making you a victim really is not. They are in service to you by creating for you the reality that you require, that you have created with your thought forms.

You are always a creator of your lives, my friends. You are never a victim. The Loving Law of Allowance allows space for all things to be in their own time and place. Non-judgment, my friends, is a key to greater understanding, to a higher vibration, to allowing all people to live their lives as *they believe them to be*, not *as you believe them to be*. It also allows you to live your life as you are, as you see it, as you believe it to be.

Love yourself; accept totally all that you are, where you are and why you are, for you are who you are because that was your need, that was your choice before incarnating. That does not mean that you must remain in that projection for the rest of your life, but it does mean that until you learn to love yourself and accept who and what you are, until you have learned the lesson that you came to learn in that particular circumstance, you are not going to move forward.

You are, my friends, on a quest for the Higher Self. You are on a quest to return to that knowing of the spiritual nature that you truly are, and to remember that you are truly *one with all life*. You are not separate. It is the physical body that gives an illusion of separateness which is not reality.

There are no problems in life, there are only events and circumstances. It is the subconscious projection, the intellect, the mind that creates the problems out of those events. This is not to say that intellect is wrong, as it has its place within your life. Otherwise you would not choose to have such a vibration to deal with. There is the

31

physical, the emotional and the mental within the physical dimension. And you're here to work with them all and to balance them into the spiritual until you are connected again with the higher source.

Taulmus

The time has come to lift yourselves from the so-called negative attitudes that you have made manifest in your lives and in your world. *Forgive* yourselves and move into the light of the higher understanding that you, in truth, are creative Gods. You have read that thought is the creative force that manifests. It is a truth, even though at times it seems to take longer to surface here in the physical. However, all thought does create, on some level, whether it is in probable worlds, past or future lives, or by coming forth as a condition that one contemplates in the present.

5

Evolutionary Cycles

Dr. Peebles

Let me remind you that the evolutionary processes on the planet Earth affect not only the human beings, but the plants, animals, and the planet itself. Not only are all the physical and tangible elements affected, but all of the invisible levels as well. The life on the planet, as well as the life in the planet (yes, within the Earth) IS affected. The process of evolution is interconnected totally with all life; therefore, that which affects one human being also affects all life forces, all life elements. There is not *one illness* that manifests that cannot be traced to the growth, the evolution of all species, all minerals, all plants, and all energies upon the planet Earth.

Now, let us take a look at that which you call AIDS. This exists, not only on this planet, but on others as well. And it is not new upon this planet or in this era. It can be traced to other times and places; however, it was not known as AIDS because your medical technologies and the scientific evolutionary developments were not capable of adequately defining so many of these viruses and infections. I would say that AIDS is more obvious now and it is being more clearly defined.

It is epidemic of nature; an epidemic which is going to continue for a long period of time. It is many years before the cure is to be found. By the time the cure is found, the virus itself will have gone through another mutation so it will not be as deadly nor confining. At this

33

point the virus will affect on still another level. The next evolutionary growth of the AIDS virus will not be an epidemic nature as it is in the current era.

This illness coincides with the cycle of evolution that our planet is going through. There is presently a major era shift taking place, from the Piscean Age to the Aquarian Age. People are actually calling upon major configurations so that life will have the *need* to evolve from the Piscean intellectual attitude into the Aquarian spiritual/mental self, the Higher Self as opposed to the personality, ego/self manifestation.

Also, at this time, there is a major grid alignment occurring within the planet, and it is approaching a major shift of the axis. This vibration has not been on the planet, at this level, for nearly 11,000 years. That calls for a major cleansing process. The appearance of this illness does not mean that humans have failed in the eyes of God. It is because there is need of cleansing. Many souls need it for their fulfillment. Yes, they need it! They *chose* to come into this lifetime for it. They chose bodies that would be exposed to the illness. They chose bodies that would be able to incubate it, that would be able to transfer it, that would be able to manifest to the degree of illness and even transition, that you would call "death."

Now here is an important point: each and every living human being has the AIDS virus within them. Each and every living being transfers that virus to others on a daily basis. Many of those who have it, in fact the mass majority, never have any symptoms. Many people to whom it is transferred, on a daily basis, will never have symptoms from it. Their natural genetic instincts reject it and counteract it. If your souls chose bodies that would automatically reject it, you do not need it. You will not experience it even if you were to have direct and living contact with an overt carrier of the powerful AIDS virus in its negative manifestation.

I am also suggesting that in this cleansing process, those bodies who have the illness, those bodies who become carriers, those bodies that make the transition, it is for them little more than giving their souls the opportunity for *their* evolutionary process. It is also part of the collective growth of the planet, for it must be cleansed. The planet must lose much of its population and it will be accomplished not only through this illness, but also through many Earth upheavals, through geographical shifts, and related occurrences.

I am suggesting that the human being intellect, the human being ego, is overreacting to a natural evolutionary process that they chose to be part of. Many of those who are saying, "Oh, I am frightened. Oh, I'm alone. Oh, I'd better look out for this," are actually counteracting their natural, instinctive immunity system to the virus. And they are calling upon this illness when it isn't even theirs. This activates a stronger element of the intensity of this illness and its manifestation.

Every living human being has the AIDS virus in them, just as they have the cancer virus. And AIDS is little more than a mutation of the existing cancer that each and every one of you have within your bodies. Other life forms, animals, and plants have the AIDS virus. AIDS is transferred, not only through human contact, through the salivas or mucous membranes, but also is transferred through all proteins. Viruses existing within proteins that are actively manifesting the infection's quality are able to transfer cancer, AIDS, etc. You would find this true of protein in red or white flesh, including fish. AIDS and cancer are found to be transferred through the protein in certain vegetables as well. There are minerals, some even that are used in building materials, some that are used as jewelry and adornments, that carry some of these viruses and are able to infect other living beings.

Dear ones, AIDS is *nothing new*. It is an ancient illness that is only more clearly definable and is only more overt at this point because of the shift of energy that you are experiencing on the planet Earth. There is no major cure to be found for AIDS *at this point* because it is a soul experience, individually and collectively. It is a natural evolutionary process and so it will not be cured before it has gone about its natural cycle and done what it was designed to accomplish.

AIDS is not something to fear. It is something to recognize as little more than another opportunity for certain souls to be fulfilled. If you look back on all of the great plagues or the great wars, you would see that they were elements that led us to evolutional consciousness. The same will be true of AIDS in retrospect.

35

Soli

The Earth goes through changes every seven or eight thousand years. The last was Noah's flood. The one before that is now mythically recorded as the Garden of Eden, and the loss of the civilization of Atlantis. The one you are headed into right now will be of much less severity than usual for so many are working upon themselves upon the Earth plane.

The Earth is moving into its reincarnation and has decided that it no longer wants to be the playground for juvenile delinquents and is going to have a much happier group of individuals on its surface. And for those who want to remain as juvenile delinquents, another planet will be of service and provide them that service.

As we say so often, society here on Earth is changing, and will continue to change. Those who wish to be a part of it will, and those who do not wish to be a part of it will not.

II

Communicating
With
The Universe

"My friends, we do not have all the answers and we do not pretend to have them. We simply bring you our perspective from a different point of view. It is rather like we are standing on the mountaintop and you are only halfway up. We can see more of the valley below than you can. Our vision is more far-reaching.... What we are trying to do is to bring certain subjects, vast knowledge, understanding and greater vision down to you in a form that your minds can accept, understand and work with."

1

What Are Spirit Guides And Teachers?

Soli

Guides and Teachers, my friends, are just that. They come in various shapes and forms. There are groups of entities that you choose to incarnate with. Some of your friends stay behind in the Spirit realm to help guide you. Many of you have been Guides and Teachers for others on the Earth plane while you were within the Spirit dimension. You are simply reversing the roles. It is as if God has split Himself up into many small parts as smaller Gods in order to experience the power of His own creation. You are one of those parts. Therefore, there is no one higher or lower than any other part of God. All creation and those in it are parts of God. There are, however, entities on different levels of evolution. Some are on a higher level because they have lived more lives and have attained more wisdom and understanding. These entities can assist you through their deeper understanding. We are called Spirit Guides. My friends, we do not have all the answers and we do not pretend to have them. We simply bring you our perspective from a different point of view.

It is rather like we are standing on the mountain top and you are only halfway up. We can see more of the valley below than you can. Our vision is more far-reaching. Whatever we believe, that is *our* interpretation. In fact, we are being taught by entities who have even greater understanding than we do. There are some who are like birds and have an *even greater* vision. What we are trying to do, however, is to bring certain subjects, vast knowledge, understanding, and greater vision down to you in a form that your minds can accept, understand, and work with subconsciously.

Also, there are very evolved, high Teachers who remain with you for your entire life. They work with you in enabling you to acquire a deeper knowledge and greater understanding in life and they guide you in many ways. But it is only guidance. No guide will ever interfere with your life. No guide will ever do anything within your life that will change your probability pattern. A guide can *lead you through a darkened room to a light switch, but he cannot make you turn it on*. That is entirely up to you by your own free will and choice.

You will notice there are many different opinions within the Spirit dimension. In this publication itself, you will find different Spirit communicators and Teachers who are bringing forward different perspectives. They are perspectives, different points of view, and as such, all have validity.

Enid

One important bridge between this Universe and the rest of life is spanned by our Spirit Guides and Teachers. Spirit Guides are only friends from the Spirit world. They are not in a body and they are most probably only in the vicinity of this plane and not a part of it. We chose them before taking a body and shared our life plans and goals with them, as well. They have promised to help us by inspiring us to attain these goals. Teachers are Spirit Guides who have agreed to assist us more specifically in areas concerning our reawakening, healing, and the arts. It is not the purpose of any of these Guides to usurp our free will or our abilities to discover enlightenment on our own. Teachers very often communicate to us in our sleep, as do all our Guides. When we are in reverie or sleep, we are most receptive to their communications. Why we need Spirit Guides, especially if we are here to stand upon our own feet and learn these lessons, is here answered.

Due to the overwhelming beliefs which have accumulated across time, as we know it, our awareness, as a species, has dwindled to small peepholes, visible to a few. There have always been those who seemed to be able to see above the clouds. They are either nearing the fulfillment of their goals here, or they have come purposefully at specific times to help inspire others to look and see what is there beyond the confines of this plane. It is never accidental, just as your own growth is never accidental. Our Guides don't try to answer all our questions for us or try to solve all our problems as much as they help us *contact our own inner selves*. In other words, they validate our own abilities to find answers for ourselves. They guide us to our own beingness. That is what is meant by guiding. It does not mean that guardian angels swoop down and keep us from getting hurt or killed. This is why we often feel we know what our Guides are going to tell us.

Gently, and with great care, they direct us to our own being so that we gain in the power of our own knowing. If the answer seems foreign or new, it only points to how far we have strayed from our own inner beingness.

It is those who are more aware who bear the responsibility of encouraging others to see. It is the burden of the more aware to be understanding and compassionate with those who are not ready to look beyond the game of this plane to the wonders in store for all of us. Spirit Guides work directly through you and through others who are more aware, to help you open up to the real realities. (Real realities describe realities outside this limited Universe. Many of the real realities are reachable in some fashion, through greater insight, awareness and growth.) Those who are more aware are not without their problems. They must grant rightness to those who would invalidate their realities in favor of those with which they are familiar; realities which are measurable, visible, touchable, and physical. At the same time, many such people talk of flying by the seat of their pants and having that old gut feeling about something and never even realize that they, too, are seeing.

41

Kyros

Sometimes you hear statements from others in which they credit their actions to spiritual guidance. Such statements are, "I have received guidance to do this or that," or "My spiritual guidance has directed me to take this action." Listening, you may wonder how one really knows if the guidance is accurate or not, or where it's coming from.

True spiritual guidance will *always* direct you into loving actions; it will never direct you into actions of non-love. If your direction guides you into actions which create pain and suffering for others, then the ego-self is in some way involved. This is the *only* test of the accuracy of guidance. It is true that pain or hurt cannot be experienced by a human entity unless that entity chooses to allow it. This truth might cause you to believe, then, that you bear no responsibility when your actions do cause pain to others. If you are aware enough to know that one allows the pain in his life experience, you should also be aware enough to know that if you consciously know your actions will cause pain to another, you must assume a degree of responsibility for the suffering caused. The metaphysical laws must never be used as a way of rationalizing your own action.

A part of awareness training is concerned with becoming attuned to the varied and differing levels of awareness within others. If you are truly aware, you must know that you are not *off the hook* if you know that your actions will cause pain for another and you proceed by thinking, "Well, if he is hurt, that's his problem. He is allowing it." This is using metaphysics to rationalize your actions. And if you must rationalize your actions, then it is improbable that the actions originated from spiritual direction.

Oftentimes, human entities use metaphysical laws as a way of rationalizing all their actions by saying they are the result of spiritual guidance, when in fact, they are prompted by ego guidance. This rationalization may be used so frequently to justify their actions that they actually come to believe that they are always operating under spiritual direction. Again, Spirit never directs an entity into actions in which the entity consciously knows he will produce suffering.

42

You cannot consciously know that your action will hurt another unless you are aware of the awareness level of the other person. In your more intimate connections with others you generally are aware of their awareness levels. Thus, you have a conscious knowledge of when your actions will cause pain. In the resultant incurring of karma, the balancing occurs not because of the pain caused to another, but because of your conscious knowledge that your action would cause pain. The one who experiences the pain does allow it and is responsible for it. The one who consciously knows he will cause pain to another is likewise responsible for that.

If you are driving down the street and you see a pedestrian and you feel directed to hit him, he will allow the experience of pain. But you, as the directed driver, consciously know or have the awareness that your hitting him will cause pain. You come under the law and you cannot rationalize or justify your action by simply saying, "Well, he is choosing to experience pain." This extreme example was given to graphically describe what occurs in more subtle life situations.

The degree of balancing is always based on intent. As you can imagine, if you plan and prepare to hurt someone, the balancing is more intense. Doing this is definitely not the result of spiritual guidance, but of ego guidance. Consciously knowing that you will hurt someone because of your knowledge of his awareness level incurs a lesser degree of karmic balancing, but again it is unlikely that it was prompted by spiritual guidance. No karma is incurred if hurt is created in another in a situation where you had neither intent nor conscious knowledge that your action would produce hurt. Humorously, the idea that "what you don't know won't hurt you" is true.

One thing you must realize is that you cannot evaluate the feelings and reactions of another by how you would react and feel in a similar situation. You should never measure another against yourself. This is just another way of rationalizing. You can't say, "Well, if this happened to me, I certainly wouldn't feel hurt. There's just no logical reason for it. So, it's his problem." Remember that feelings are seldom based on logic and what you feel or do not feel is *unique to you* .

Essentially, then, spiritual guidance comes from a point of love and directs the entity into loving actions designed to promote the highest good. Anything less than this must be analyzed carefully. If actions must be rationalized, using metaphysical laws or anything else, they do not originate from spiritual guidance. True spiritual guidance never needs to be justified or rationalized to yourself or others. If you consciously know that your action will cause pain to another because of your knowledge of his awareness level and you still proceed, then you assume responsibility for that knowing and must be prepared for balancing.

Spirit *always* leads one toward attunement with the varied and differing awareness levels of others. And, finally, Spirit always seeks to direct the entity to his greatest unfoldment and lovingly directs that entity into actions promoting the highest growth and unfoldment for all within his individual world.

2

Channeling And Mediumship

Dr. Peebles

All living beings, human, plants, or animals are channels of energy and vibration. All living things are vessels that allow the Universal Mind, God, to flow into them. Even the plants channel the Universal God energy. Animals channel ideas, inspiration, healing. Human beings channel light, inspiration, healing.

All things have lived, all things live. Part of you is in the plant right now. Part of every animal is existing within you right now. All of your past lives, all of your future lives are in you, right now. When you have recall of another life, when you have deja vu, you are channeling, bringing through a recall vibration of what you once were, or what you will be. When you become aware that another person is going to call you on the telephone, you are channeling the telepathic communication. You have telepathically been in touch with that person, and have created, collectively, a communication that was not physical. Both of you have channeled the spirit of communication.

Channeling is not just bringing the words and guidance from the spirit world. Channeling is sharing ideas, inspiration, love, and power. Channeling is of healing, right action, joy, laughter, inspiration. Channeling is the manifestation of the non-physical planes into the physical density, bringing the other dimensions and realms into the physical, flowing through the vortex of the provided body. All of

45

those things existing in the Universe are available to each of you, for they are in you. Channeling is when you open yourself up and remove yourself from the intellectual to such a degree that those other dimensions are able to manifest.

Now there are *levels* of channeling, of course. That does not mean that any of the levels are *better* than the others. Deep trance, light trance, conscious, whatever; they're *all* channeling, admitting something exists beyond their own intellectual control. The majority of channels are conscious, and in their consciousness they influence and filter much that is being inspired. Even those who are deep trance mediums influence and filter, just to a lesser degree. It is for you to see that to be alive, you are a channel of the Spirit. The Spirit is not out there alone, *it is in you!*

Soli

Understand that which is termed mediumship. Mediums are those able to center the subconscious mind, to reduce it to its smaller part, in order to allow the communication from the Higher Self to come through. What you are seeking to do is the same thing. Every single individual upon the Earth plane is a medium, one who communicates. A person who channels spoken words from one who is in the Spirit dimension is but one form, one structure, which is neither better nor worse, higher nor lower than any other form of mediumship. You are a medium in whatever you do in your life.

If you are happy and joyful, if you feel fulfilled in what you are doing, then you are the highest medium you can be, for you are doing what you need to do without worrying about what others are telling you to do. You are communicating joy and happiness to others through your actions in life. You emit those vibrations which others can feel and pick up. You become a medium for those vibrations. For example, you happen to pass an ordinary street sweeper who is happy, joyful and whistles all day long while he is sweeping away. He is thoroughly enjoying himself, not wishing for something else, not judging himself to be lower than anyone else because of his job. You will actually feel a lift from that energy, and, in fact, be healed from

46

that medium who is sweeping the street! This is truly what medium-ship is.

Kyros

Because each entity is individually connected to the Universal Mind, channeling is occurring all of the time at some level. Universal Thought flows into individualized mind, which is composed of the various levels of consciousness. You are all aspects of the collective consciousness, individual droplets of water in the vast ocean of Universal Mind. You have access to all information stored there, you need only to learn how to tune in and listen. All that pours forth from Universal Mind is pure and designed for the highest good of all creation. A Universal Thought, however, loses some of its purity as it moves through the levels of consciousness.

You must remember that Universal Thought is an energy which can never be accurately deciphered and interpreted by the human brain computer. You must also remember that what is verbalized by the human channel is influenced to a degree by the channel's own programming, his ego, his level of awareness, his collective consciousness. There is no pure human channeling. Probably the purest thoughts one has are those which cannot be verbalized, and you all have many of those. As a human channel grows and expands in awareness and becomes more consciously aligned to the Universal Mind, the channeling is less influenced by these things.

What I want you to understand is that which is termed "channeling" is not a unique phenomenon. Everyone channels whether they call it that or not. So, when someone says this or that was "channeled," it does not necessarily mean that it is to be *your* truth. All you have on planet Earth is relative truth, and what is true for one may not be so for another. You must test all input from your external world against your own sense of truth. The human entity should still learn to test another's truth against his own and to become connected to his own higher guidance. Some entities depend on channels to tell them what to do in their lives or to tell them what will happen in the future. Some channels do have the awareness to give the answers to you, and sometimes, they can predict a future with great accuracy. Most, however, are adept at reading probabilities based on an awareness of a present state of consciousness.

You are ever-changing, and with a mere shift in consciousness, you can alter your life course. Psychics have a great awareness of human patterns, and they predict probabilities based on the present consciousness. And each one of you can do this for yourselves by simply becoming aware and attuned to your own present consciousness.

Your highest guidance is uniquely for you and it is the only guidance you should trust completely. You have all your own answers, and even though your answers may help others as well, they are still yours.

Enid

Channeling is the result of surrendering with the certain knowledge that a being or beings are communicating from another plane and that we can bring that communication into the physical Universe through our own minds and bodies and relate those communications to ourselves and to others. These communications can come through as intuition, as a certain *feeling* about an event, be it past, present or future; they can come through in the forms of inner, silent, or audible sounds or in the form of inner, visible words or pictures. These descriptions are made in this manner in order to describe almost impossible-to-describe concepts concerning the receipt of communications from other realms. Communications can come through the mouth as words without any perception of the form that sent it. They can come through when we write (without thinking) in our notebooks after asking questions. They rarely come without our invitation, although they have been known to impinge upon us, asking us to receive them.

No matter in what form they come, they are sometimes easy to deny. They are soft, often subtle, and feel much as though we are thinking them on our own. Perhaps the biggest problem is in letting the communication stand for itself and acknowledging it. Once you have, you will love it. You will feel great joy when you channel. The degree and quality of that kind of sharing is so beautiful and fulfilling that you will soon lose all possible doubt as to its reality in truth.

3

Communicating With Spirits

Ting-Lao

I have heard beings comment about what if there really is an "other side," and what if one can talk with the dead and have the dead talk through them, and of what use it is. Such communications are useful, not only to gain knowledge, but to make your life work better for you. Many times people hold onto it as simply more knowledge, and do not use it in their daily lives as practical information.

When you have a problem and don't know what to do, you confide in people who care about you and ask them for their help. You sometimes call these people angels, these people who are good and loving. There are those on the spirit side who do not possess bodies but who are looking for ways to help, who want to do something and have something to offer. They cannot offer, as it is not their right to meddle or interfere, without an invitation, in a life that is not their own. But, if you ask them for help, then it is a different story. They are very glad to have something constructive and helpful to do.

I am saying in general, then, that you people can ask those on the "other side" to help in certain situations in which you do not know what else to do or how to handle them, just as you would ask a friend on this side. It is a little different than praying to God, because some of us are seen as messengers of God. There is an old Indian saying that when the Christians would say, "Jesus is the Son of God, the messenger of God," the Indians would say, "Would God underestimate the problem so much that He would only send one helper?" Well, you can see the Spirit people as helpers or messengers of God. And when one specifically asks for their help, it is beneficial to both.

Soli

Many souls have had great experiences within the Earth plane, the Earth dimension, and have great love for it. Such entities recognize, once they have left the Earth plane, the growth, the change, the experiences, the beauty that they have had within the Earth plane. They recognize that the way forward for *all* entities is to learn that they are God, that the way lies *within and not without*.

And so, they, out of great love, decide and choose to work with channels, bringing forward greater knowledge, greater energy within the physical dimension. There are some who choose such a task for the difficulty of it, rather out of challenge to see how they can effect change upon the Earth plane without directly interfering, how they can bring forward information, energy, and knowledge.

Understand that we can only work if the energy is attractive enough to draw those who would wish to listen, and so there is challenge within that. This is part of our growth and experience and evolution to learn to work in this way.

Those of us within the Spirit dimension who are teaching in this way, through channels, are not single Spirits, are not individuals, although we do use names like Soli or Dr. Peebles, etc. We choose a personality by which to be known, to present the energy to those within the physical dimension. If we were to present ourselves in our present vibrational state, you would not be able to withstand the energy.

And so we choose, as a transformer of our own energy, a lifetime that one particular spiritual entity has had. The energy of those who are teaching is transformed, as it were, into a lower vibrational level so that it can be perceived safely by those of similar vibrational level within the physical dimension.

Master Adalfo

There *are* such beings as angels. They are great-light bearers. It is a lovely thought to believe in Guardian Angels. It is even true. You have these beings of light who are always around you to shed light for you when you feel that you are in darkness. You can ask them to help you by saying, "Please send me a 100-watt light bulb now because I am feeling like I am in darkness."

Many people are wondering why communication with Spirits has increased recently. It seems that many people are now involved with this at this time. However, there has always been communication with the Spirit dimension. You see, as the planet evolves, people also evolve. The more evolved people there are on the planet at one time, the more apparent this communication becomes. Right now, there are, indeed, many who are highly evolved on Earth.

Enid

Even though we describe various ways of communicating with Spirits, your own experience will be unique. There are several major ways in which we can communicate, but these are not, by any means, the only ones. We repeat: there is *nothing cut and dried about the Spirit world.* Communication can be done directly, through telepathy. It comes through as thought and *feels* mostly as though it were your own. The minute we get a surprising bit of data, we know for certain that it isn't coming from us. It may come as though it is a memory and may be that shadowy, but it can be trusted. One is in a light trance, here. We call it *open* channeling or conversational channeling.

It can also be done through writing or automatic writing. You can sit with pen and paper, thinking or writing down a question. Words will instantly come to mind. Do not throw them away, but write them down. Trust them. Allow yourself to get over any feeling of self-consciousness. Let come what comes. Eventually, you will find yourself writing faster than you could compose sentences in your own mind. Do not bother to evaluate what is coming to you. This will stop

52

the flow and is an invitation to filter. The hardest answers to write down are those that fit what we thought that answer might be or what we thought it should be; or if the answers flatter us, we tend to discount them as wishful thinking. You can rest assured that such is not the case. We, as a species, tend to *disavow* good things said about us or to us about ourselves.

Channeling can be done through a deeper trance. You can open yourself up and allow communication to come through, using your own body as a vehicle for the guide. Many times a guide will use the name and some aspects of personality very similar to the last physical existence, or, in some cases, a favorite one. Beings are not really gender-oriented when out of physical form, although they will generally project themselves as though they are male or female.

Some mediums are conscious of the messages coming through them and some go into a deeper trance state for fear of filtering or shedding bias on the messages being received. Most mediums or channels are careful to a fault to communicate exactly what is being transmitted.

There are degrees of channeling in this manner. It varies from a light trance, in which the channel's own voice and accent is used, to deeper trance states, in which the guide speaks with a totally different sound and accent and, of course, to all possible degrees that exist between. If you allow a being to speak through you, your voice, accent and type of language will probably be different, even if barely perceptible, from yours. This is true, especially in deeper trance states. It can also be true if you are channeling while still in a conscious state. You can listen in, so to speak. You can understand, however, that you are still a part of the communication, even while in deep trance. We call this direct channeling. The Spirits come through directly as themselves. Many call this transmediumship, or trance channeling.

That also requires practice. Your Guides depend upon your vocabulary and your understanding while channeling through you, so don't be surprised to hear colloquial phrases and expressions from time to time. This does not indicate negative filtering at all. We are not empty shells. But you can also realize that the part of you that enters itself into the communication is your finest, most impartial self. Trust it.

We also communicate with our Guides and others every time we sleep. We can learn to be conscious of this communication and to decipher our dreams. We can go to bed and establish firmly, with concentration, those things about which we wish to be enlightened. Then, while we are out of the body and are freely conversing with our friends, we can work on ideas and concepts that we want to know more about or that we want to unravel. Our dreams, however, when we can remember them, come cloaked in the symbols of this Universe. Most of the time we can figure them out.

One thing is for certain, that others will probably not be able to figure them out for us, since symbols are mostly personal choices. Our Guides can help us, however. They can help us to be inspired by our dreams. The reason others find it difficult to translate our dreams is that a river, for instance, may signify great freedom for one person and a fear of death to another. Sometimes, the obvious is not always true.

As we said before, there are other ways in which we communicate, and once we open up to any of those ways, we can open up to the others. We can channel music, poetry, songs, dance, painting, drawing, architecture, design anything at all. We can channel it by inspiration, or directly, by allowing ourselves to surrender to another's direction, thus sharing in the creation. After having successfully channeled our friends for a good long period of time, we will notice that we are sharing conceptual thought and telepathic understanding without employing the usual methods of communication. This is a very high level of communication and greatly desired among our friends. When this happens, it signals success in reaching closely into our inner being, our inner knowing. The time for seeking advice is nearing an end, and channeling from your own inner being has expanded, opened a new way of expanding the awareness. Awareness expands to the degree that we are able to connect with our inner beingness.

Being able to trust our own knowingness is *vital* to our growth. When we are channeling from our inner being, we are tapped into All

There Is. This does not mean that we are finished with our Guides. They are closer than ever at this point.

Visionary communication also occurs. We can develop the ability to see physical manifestations of beings, if they are, indeed, there. There are beings who are highly evolved enough and interested in the physical Universe enough to show themselves in some kind of physical form. Failure to see one does in no way lessen the other forms of communication. We stress this because there are many who are innocently ignoring great and wondrous communications only because they cannot *see* anything.

We really do not need to depend upon the physical Universe to reassure us that the Spirit world exists. We can simply *know* that it does. It needs no physical proof of its existence. The painting does not have to *prove* that it was created by something outside itself. It also doesn't have to prove that it takes something or someone outside itself to realize that it exists, yet it is true. Those who need such proof of the existence of the Spirit and of beings without bodies who can communicate with us are not ready to know, and no amount of reasoning will convince them. It is true that only those who are ready to know have experienced visionary communications. Remember that true vision comes with understanding, not in seeing with the eyes.

III

The Meaning Of Disease

"The Higher Self will try to get you back on track, if you are off course. It will try to move you into a direction in order for you to have those experiences that you wanted. How does it do this? The Higher Self must communicate with you. It does this through illness.

The key to getting beyond the communication of disease, which is the lack of ease, is to follow your intuition, follow your inner guidance.

You will have the most ease when you are doing that.

If you followed the guidance of the Higher Self continually, without thought, without question, without fear, without doubt, you would never be ill in your life."

1

Epidemics

Enid

Let's look at our society as a whole. We have what we call epidemics. This is when a whole army of beings decides to experience something together. So, they all have the flu and they say, "Did you get that, too?" You see, it's a point of connection. Wars also cause a point of connection. People say, "Are you afraid? I am, too. Let's talk about it, let's get together." Perhaps they never spoke with each other before.

Whenever there is an epidemic, there is a common experience in which the whole society seems to come out a little bit better afterwards than they were before. After having a flu, do you remember how clean inside you felt? You're just so clean. Sometimes an illness has helped you to start over in some way, to cleanse you.

When you have the flu or a very bad cold, or some other illness, you get rid of all your toxins, which come out of your body. Your body just flushes and flushes itself out. The more liquids you take the more your body is flushed. When it is over, you feel weak, like a new calf, but you feel so clean inside. It's really true that your body and all its cells are beginning to rejuvenate and you can help it by good diet and good thoughts about the body and by loving it more. You can say, "Now that you're all clean, let's start something new, some new project or something." Something good always happens after an illness, that you'll notice.

Sometimes a whole country can experience this same type of cleansing process. The great plagues were ways of helping beings who had been coming back too long in the same place. Plagues always happened in overcrowded areas such as London, in those early days. If you remember, there was so much crowding and so many people living together, with excrement in the streets and everything was so dirty and unclean. Plagues gave cities a chance to start over, a chance to breathe with fewer people. It also made people aware of doing something about keeping their streets clean. Then the consciousness about cleanliness began to be raised.

Dong How Li

There were catastrophic diseases before in human history, but they were not called AIDS; they were called other things. One in the last century was called consumption. The human body has reached a level now where it requires larger masses of disease within it to fell it. The body has progressed biologically with regard to its ability to fight off certain diseases. Now the psyche and the physicality of the human body has *upped the ante*, and this is a new game called AIDS. There have always been plagues. This is a new plague with a new name. It is no different. Ultimately all plagues attack the same system which is the immune system.

The Great Plague physicalized Christian repression and the subsequent government repression at that time. Repression always follows an age of expansion, just as disease does. Disease followed the "Great Flowering," the Renaissance, as well as the Inquisition in the early 1100's. That plague physicalized what was going on in the value structures of the time, as manifested in political oppression. The same thing is happening now. Only in this case, where sexuality is concerned, AIDS is the restriction after the flowering of sexual liberation in the sixties.

The challenge of it is for each and every one of you, starting with those who have it and then those in concentric circles beyond them, to find responsibility *now* in the freedom to have sex, to move up from the first chakra and engage the heart at the fourth chakra. You are

60

going to find people putting condoms back on, while in the sixties, they had taken them off, as well as their bras and briefs.

Master Adalfo

Diseases change over the years, as you know, and different ones come to the forefront. On Atlantis, we had diseases, not exactly the same diseases as today, but different ones that were appropriate to the time and place, in order to teach us what we were needing to know. There were similar issues then, of course. However, they were slightly different in the sense that there was greater knowledge then. People wanted to possess all of God's knowledge as their own. They wanted personal power over God's knowledge. They had great mental powers then (which you do not have now), and they were trying to use them to take over from God. They wanted to be in charge. So, the diseases we had were a little bit different. They were diseases about power and the use of power.

If we talk about things at their highest level, you will see there is a similarity between AIDS and the plague. With the plague, there was an issue of power, of wanting power which people did not have. Different diseases manifest at different times to illustrate the same lesson in a new ways. You do not have the actual plague now because it would not have the same effect, particularly since you would know what to do about it.

Ting-Lao

Let me say a little bit about the catastrophic effects that this illness will have on humanity, since AIDS is a plague in proportion to the bubonic plague. These ancient diseases have formed their "entityness" on the culture of humanity. They have left big scars on the continuum of humanity throughout time, and energy does not travel through a scar well. It is, therefore, very important for each person in the culture to learn from the disease, now. Each person in the culture needs to be learning even though they do not know anyone who has AIDS, or even if they think that they will not meet anyone

61

who has AIDS. It is important not to deny that it is happening in the world, in the human culture.

It is important to again wake up and realize what is happening to all the people because you are all bonded in many ways, in energy ways. You must learn from the disease now because later it will become encapsulated, just like the bubonic plague. You do not know much about that plague, but it was a catastrophic time of changes for the people in humanity. Whole gene pools were destroyed. It is important to learn the knowledge of the gene pools that were changed, altered and destroyed, just as it is important to seek out and help the people who have this illness, or any illness.

Now is the time before it becomes encapsulated in history. Do it now, so that humanity does not have to continue having these epidemics. Do it now so that people will again raise their consciousness and their awareness of the possibilities of life with new understanding and knowledge. Do it now so you will learn in easier ways instead of learning in such hard ways.

2

Why Illness?

Your Need For Experience

Dr. Peebles

My friends, strive diligently not to understand where an illness came from, nor where it is going. Do not attempt to justify why you or another have any illness, be it a broken bone, cancer, or AIDS. Recognize that it is an experience that is there for you at that moment or you would not be aware of it. Recognize that it is not for you to justify or to fear. It is only for you to accept it so totally that you are able to elevate it to its highest possible soul experience, for yourself and for others as well.

Do not even consider that you have done anything wrong nor anything that puts you aside from acceptance by the Spirit Guides or from God. Recognize that you, as a soul, are experiencing an event and you have a decision to make. Will you live it in the Earth-binding webs and shadows or will you live it on a higher level for all to observe that there are other alternatives. Will you, by your actions, show others that they have the ability to lift their reactions to a higher level? Those who cannot accept you for whatever illness or manifestation you have, that becomes *their* problem, not *yours*. Your only problem is to take your experience and elevate it to the highest level so that everyone around you will say, "If they are able to accomplish it, then I, too, may be able to accomplish it."

There are so many people who are saying, "I'm being very good right now. I'm not having any intravenous drugs. I am not having indiscriminate sex, therefore, I am not going to get AIDS." My friends, if your soul intended it in the first place, then you will get it through a vegetable or a fish.

Remember that when the soul leaves its perfect state and begins the cycles of birth and death, in its karmic interchange it develops the need for certain experiences. Illness often is little more than the tool to give the soul the opportunity to balance itself. Even if you are a highly evolved vibration or soul, you still have the need to be around the environment, to see illnesses. Frequently, you will have an illness. You can use your illness as an opportunity to transcend, to move back onto the Spirit plane. If you hold on, you will build new karma, which then creates the need for new balance. Illness, then, on the higher plane, is little more than a tool to accomplish a specific goal, to return to the light. *Illness is not something that God levies upon you. Illness is an experience that God allows you to use in your soul's evolution.*

Soli

The Higher Self does not know negativity. All it wants is experiences. The Higher Self might very well decide, "Hmmmm, pain is one of the aspects of life within the physical body. I've never experienced it to any great extent. I need to have a lifetime that is full of pain. I will choose a body, parents, with a very strong, dogmatic belief system that will be almost impossible to ignore." And that belief system will keep that individual from following the inner guidance. That will create pain and it will be experienced.

The Higher Self, however, does not know pain. In the spiritual dimension you do not know pain and suffering; it does not exist. It is part of the subconscious, its beliefs and its resistance to change. The Higher Self is trying to move you into following its guidance.

Enid

If you take a look at it, the whole idea of a *dreadful illness* is a very

64

exciting thing. And if you'll notice, there's really no good or bad experience, it's all just experience. Some experiences we enjoy more than others. When we go back home to the Spirit plane we look back and say, "You know, that dreadful time after I broke my hip, it was so dreadful, but I have to tell you that when I look back at that time, I see so many glories there, so many things I learned to understand."

There are things that cannot be understood with sweetness and light because that's what we have *outside* this Universe. So, we come here and grit our teeth and say, "Okay, sock it to me. I'll take it. I will take whatever it is you want to dish out because I want to experience it." So, you're sitting here with sympathetic thoughts toward yourself and others who are suffering dire things. Well, where else can you experience that? Where else can you experience getting robbed if you don't invite a robber in? Where else can you experience an automobile wreck unless you're driving an automobile? All these experiences create enormous energy within us.

Lack of Communication With Your Higher Self

Soli

Your physical bodies are microcosms of the macrocosmic Earth. Every molecule that exists upon the Earth exists within your body. Every single germ imaginable, and a large number of germs unimaginable to medical science, are already in your physical body. They are there. It is not that you *catch* them from someone else. It is that you lay yourself open, by your thoughts, to having the germs multiply. Every single illness that you can imagine is already inside you. If you do not worry about them, if you do not need that communication, then they do not need to manifest.

Indeed, these germs are in service to you, my friends. They are giving you communications of the *need* to change. That is the important point. Whenever you find yourself being ill, ask yourself, "What is it in my life that I am doing that is creating this? What is the *communication?* What do I need to change? What have I done over these last few weeks? What thoughts have I had about myself? Have

65

I been feeling depressed? Have I been telling myself what a terrible person I am, how untalented, how impossible it is for me to do anything? Have I been telling my body how ugly it is?"

Most people feel themselves to be victims, either victims of other people, or victims of disease, and they seek someone else to relieve them, to change it for them. So, they go to a doctor and take a few pills, anything to relieve the symptoms. But unless the communication is understood, either that same disease or another one of greater severity will come along. Sometimes the communication is never heard, and at that point, the Higher Self says, "There's not much point staying upon the Earth plane any longer as we see no probability of experiencing anything of value in this physical body. It is time to leave." So, that person contracts a terminal illness. It need not be like this, as it is the choice of the individual.

Doctors in old China only got paid if their patients were cured. Imagine the medical profession working on those terms today! Those doctors of China *understood the true nature and cause of illness*. They understood that if a husband and wife were fighting constantly, illness would manifest itself sooner or later. So, those doctors spent their time walking through the neighborhoods, talking to their patients, dealing with their problems, listening, and discovering what was causing the difficulty in their lives and helping them to change that. As long as their patients were well, they were working and were successful.

Master Adalfo

Examine why disease is in your life. Is your life unhappy or unpleasant so that disease is needed to be drawn to you in order to fix it? Because disease does *fix* something, even if only to make you ill enough to stay in bed. What is it doing for you? What does it make you look at that you never had to look at before? Ask yourself, "What changes, what growth, what evolution can I create to stop this process?" Maybe you will need help from a healer about these possible changes in your life. Then you must be willing to try them and to see what works. Experimentation with diet, exercise and even maybe

66

taking a pill from your doctor. Could be, you know, that some things can be fixed and *then* talked about.

Dong How Li

Illness, for most people, has to do with isolation. I speak both of isolation from other humans and also as in separation of various parts of their self that they are no longer in communication with. So, then, illness becomes an absence of wholeness, an absence of communication among the various parts, and that gets enacted in the physical world. So, you can understand how disease has to do with a difficulty of movement, both in the body and in the world. If one were going to begin to correct disease and go more into ease, one must begin the process of reconnection. One must face the original fears that drove one to separate.

It is what many of you are going through at other levels as is anyone whom you consider to be ill. So, the question is not only how to proceed with the reconnection, but also how to deal with all the questions, fears and shadows that it raises and how to recognize them. It is hard, when you are ill, to understand that the shadow is but a shadow. The memory and the intensity of the memory that make it all too real. If you hold the shadow in fear too long, then, indeed, it becomes real. It becomes like darkness in the body. In order to remove darkness, one brings light to it. In this case one becomes willing to take the shadow and put it in the light. Some of you make light with your hands, many of you with your eyes, and others with various kinds of touch, like embracing. It is all healing. It is truly all loving. In the loving, the reconnection is made.

You see, there is wisdom in the depths of your being that calls forth what you need, even if you choose not to invite it. If you choose to invite it, then you have already begun the process of reconnecting with the hidden parts of you. You have already begun your healing. When you invite new energy into places that are not well, they begin to feel the hurt that originally drove them into numbness. So, sometimes, the pain is the pain of awakening. It is coming back to life, coming back into wholeness. Either way you are feeling the intensity

67

of being born and of dying, of going to sleep and awakening, the impact of moving the energy.

The Need Of Attracting Your Attention

Dong How Li

Many times sickness is an invited condition. It is a way to force oneself to slow down and become conscious. It is a way to attract attention. It is also a way to totally shift one's inner and outer realities. Some of the viral diseases, particularly where fevers are concerned, can bring about this shift in one's reality.

It's like anger. It's one of those things you use to gather enough energy to move off your position in some part of your life because your culture doesn't legitimately allow you a way to do that. You are supposed to stay on your job from nine to five for 50 years with a vacation of two weeks a year. So, how do you get out of that prison? Perhaps by inviting an illness to help you activate change?

There are other prisons too: those of consciousness. Then illness becomes a way to pressurize yourself out of it. Your culture is not interested in intensity. It is interested in an *even keel with few highs and few lows.* However, if you cannot experience the intensity of the pain, how can you experience the intensity of ecstatic love? If you have no peaks, your life is all plateaus.

You wonder why there is so much burnout in your culture? Because it is all too tedious. So, one gets sick in order to break out of the tedium. I speak of the unconscious, as no one *consciously* invites disease. If you listen carefully to your own words, you can hear your words actually inviting disease to come forward.

Moving You Back On Course

Soli

If you move off your chosen course, your Higher Self will try to get you back on track. It will try to move you into a direction in order for you to have those experiences that you wanted. How does it do this? The Higher Self must communicate with you. If you followed the guidance of the Higher Self continually, without thought, without question, without fear, without doubt, you would never be ill in your life. Your body would not age because it would not *need* to age.

The Higher Self, out of love for you, out of your need, out of your agreement before incarnation, must communicate with you. It can communicate through the physical aspects, as well as the spiritual. You have the opportunity to communicate with your Higher Self through the spiritual aspects, through meditation, through understanding, through feeling. The Higher Self must communicate with you in a way that you will take notice of.

FIRST, YOUR HIGHER SELF BRINGS FORWARD AN IDEA, a thought form that you should be doing something. If you cannot understand that communication, or if you refuse to understand that communication, which happens very often, if you do not wish to hear it and willfully do not wish to go in that direction, then the Higher Self must slow the vibration down. It slows the vibration down to a stage so you receive it within the emotional body, so you *feel* the emotions regarding a circumstance, a situation you are in.

YOU BEGIN TO FEEL EMOTIONAL. You have this emotion or reaction telling you that you need to make a change in your life. Yet, very few people will understand that. Very few will take action. Most people will sit back and wonder why they are feeling so depressed, where the frustration is coming from, why that person is doing these things to me? Always the victim, looking for someone else to blame. And so they would not hear or understand that communication.

YOUR HIGHER SELF SLOWS THE VIBRATION further until it manifests within the physical body. There are very few individuals who can ignore a physical communication, be it in the form of a disease, an accident, or some physical disability. It is not easy to ignore this. When you find yourself flat on your back for a few days, you cannot ignore that situation. So, you ask yourself, "What is this communication?" Until you understand that communication from your Higher Self, there cannot be any healing. It is impossible because the *communication is the disease*.

69

It is a combination of your subconscious mind driving you in one direction and feelings and guidance wishing to take you in another direction. It is a reaction of your subconscious mind. It is resistance from the subconscious mind that causes disease. Pain and suffering exist only within the subconscious mind. They are not of spiritual origin. They are the reaction of the subconscious that refuses to follow that inner guidance, to follow that path. That is what causes disease, pain, and suffering.

Master Adalfo

Many people perceive that disease is a test of spirituality. I do not like that concept because if someone gives you a test, it implies that you should have the knowledge to pass it. So, in saying that disease is a test of spirituality, it is as if we Spirits are saying, "Well, he should have learned all this by now, we will test him by giving him a disease. See what he does with it." Obviously, this is not how we Spirits operate.

When you are ill, it is more difficult to continue to communicate with Spirit or be in touch with your own Higher Self because all of your energy goes toward staying alive or being without pain. And yet, it is an ideal time to continue your connection with Spirit so we can help you. It is true you may not have the energy to continue this connection. Realize that you can call on others to help keep you connected, even in a small way, with Spirit. In this way, you can begin to know what is going on with you and the illness.

If you talk about the good things that come from disease: it is a gift you give yourself so that you can begin to examine things more closely, so that you can begin to *feel*. With the information you have available, disease was the best gift you could come up with to make you more aware. Next time you might come up with a better present for yourself.

Ignoring Stress

Master Adalfo

Stress is a condition of imbalance, and this imbalance leads to disease, a state of being when the body is not *at ease*. Stress affects not only the physical, mental, emotional, and spiritual bodies, it also resides in the auric field around those bodies. Sometimes it can be removed by a healer before it actually attacks the physical body, just as disease can be removed from the auric field before it appears in the body.

Stress also can affect the organs in the body through a process of deterioration of wellness. An organ that is attacked by stress goes through a process that leads to gradual, slow deterioration. The attacking, caused by worry or concern, is really coming from the person, not from outside. In other words, you could have a little bit of stress in your life and you would handle it with no problem. You might decide, "I can reduce this stress by doing such and such a thing." And in this way, stress is dealt with.

However, if you have stress, and all you do is stew about it, if you take no steps, no positive action, this causes unwellness and in this way stress begins to deteriorate the organs. You may say, "Oh, I am so stressed. My job is such a problem and I don't know what to do about it." And you take no steps, all you do is worry and complain. Once stress appears in your life, whether it is your own creation or coming from factors outside of yourself, how you react to it is an *inside job*.

Kyros

Your culture seems to be over-stressed. This is due primarily to the extremely high negativity which is prevalent in your mass consciousness. A lot of methods used to relieve stress are as damaging to the physical shell and mind as stress itself. I am, of course, referring to alcohol, drugs, tranquilizers, and so on. These are illusory ways of alleviating stress and are not permanent. They

71

merely blind you for the moment.

The more positive ways of alleviating stress lie in the areas of reshaping your thinking processes and learning to control your mind, such things as self-hypnosis, muscle relaxation, centering, biofeedback, positive thinking, and so forth. A certain amount of stress is good in that it triggers you into action. You would accomplish very little if there was not some degree of stress present, for it urges you onward. This is healthy stress.

The most damaging kind of stress though is the self-created one, the stress created by the ego and its negative perceptions of the world. It is this unnatural stress which leads entities into the use of illusory methods of alleviation, and it is this type of stress which creates most of the illness (physical and mental) in your world. Each physical entity has an internal limit beyond which he cannot pass. If he goes beyond that point, the stress factor will begin its destruction of body and mind. As I look at your culture it appears that most entities have either gone beyond that point or live right on the edge of it.

When you feel or sense stress within, you need to analyze it and learn to assess whether it is natural, healthy, positive stress or whether it is manufactured stress leading to possible destruction. Worry and fear are unnatural stress, while concern and legitimate caution are healthy. In other words, you can be concerned without worrying, and you can exercise caution without experiencing fear. There's a big difference. Worry and fear are destructive types of stress.

When you feel stress, think about what is causing it. Determine how important the object causing the stress is. Can you change the circumstances by either worry or fear? Will the situation drastically alter your life? As I've told you before, most things which you deem important are not that important on a cosmic level. In fact, most things will lose their importance in a short time.

Too much energy is wasted in worry about the future and in fear of the future. If you take each moment as it comes to you, if you deal with issues as they come and then let them go, you secure your future in a more positive way.

Human life moves through time and space. You cannot stop this flow, and you will find your journey more enjoyable and positive if you start learning to analyze what is really important. Entities need to learn to become more acutely aware of their present moments in order to gain the fullness of life. This does not mean that you should not make plans or prepare for future moments. In a time/space dimension it seems that you must. You must plant the fields in spring to prepare for the autumn harvest. But you don't worry about the harvest while you're planting the seeds. You enjoy and find the pleasure in the present moment of planting the seeds. And if the locusts come and destroy the harvest, you have at least enjoyed the planting of the seeds.

The best way to be free of destructive stress is to live your present moments fully and then let them slip where they must go into the past. Stay in the present moment. You can't change past moments and you can only dream and prepare for future ones. In truth, the only moment you have a guarantee of on Earth is the one you are living. Learn to relax and do the best you can with your present moments.

Ting-Lao

Again, we need to question ourselves about why we are ill. It is due to the misalignment of energy somewhere. It is possible for you to explore this and find out in which realm of your being this energy flow is misaligned. When it is truly physical, check to see if you have too many toxins in the body, or are consuming too much sugar, caffeine or some poison. That is a misalignment that you can correct easily enough with proper diet and care of your body.

If it is an emotional misalignment, ask yourself if the reason that you don't feel the happiness around you fully is because of the fear of feeling the unhappiness also. For the pains and joys go together. Is there an emotional imbalance? Is it mental? Are you living by certain rules that are not necessarily so? Or is it spiritual? Are you having a view of your purpose in life and are you taking steps to unfold as much as possible? These are some things to contemplate when one is ill so that you can use the illness as an indicator of where the misalignment of energies is.

Living In The Fast Lane

Red Tree

All illness is a state of mind. Think about this for awhile. *All* illness is a state of mind. It is a creation of mind first. Now, I know there will be many who will say that, "I am ill due to infection. I am ill due to an accident. I am ill due to something that I did not think about." But this is not really true. You do not have to think about it with the conscious mind. I speak of a *way of thought* in life.

There are many of you on the Earth that do not believe you want illness, do not believe that you want to have an accident. But this is not the way you live, for your body expressions and even your words are contrary to this. You travel down the roadways of life in your fast automobiles, passing many things on the road, taking unnecessary risks. This is not natural.

It is the herd instinct to go over a cliff into the destruction, as a herd of cattle will do when they stampede. You people on the Earth are doing this very thing. You follow the instinct of the herd when you follow the dietary habits that are self-destructive.

There is a solution, there is a cure for you people of the world. The nature of illness is in your mind and, in your mind, there is also a cure. The cure is to have a release for this creative energy that you seek to release into the Earth but are unable to release because of the limitations imposed upon you by the society in which you find yourself.

It is that spirit of trying that I speak of. This spirit is necessary for you people on the Earth. You must have a little spirit—the spirit to try and to succeed in whatever goal you wish for yourself and also have the desire to help others in this goal. This is necessary in order to insure your success. You cannot escape the physical death of the body on the Earth. This is not possible. But you can extend it. More importantly, you can extend it with an *aura of accomplishment.*

You can have a creative life regardless of the condition you find yourself in right now. I know it is possible to be creative, even if your whole body is unable to move from a paralysis. You can create love in

74

your life. You can create beauty, as is seen in many beautiful flowers. You can see the sky even though you are blind. You can see the beauty in thought, in feeling, in life. Your awareness is the stepping stone for your creativity. Once you start creating, you will no longer be wanting to risk life and limb in your insane rush to get ahead of others. Rather, you will already be ahead.

Yes, I have seen your vehicles traveling down the highway of life. I see many people trying to pass others and, in doing so, they are always going faster, catching up with the cars in front of them and, thus, always being behind others. I think that it is wise to slow down and then you will see that others will be behind you and, in that way, you will be the leader of the roadway. More importantly, you will be the leader in life by slowing down.

You will actually be doing a thing that is natural to do. First of all, you cannot see the beautiful flowers, the trees, the grass and all the things that are not seen when you drive down the highway of life too fast. When you are walking or riding a bicycle, you can, indeed, see things that you did not know were there when you drove down the highway so fast. It is also this way in other aspects of life. When you are rushing too fast, you are overlooking the very thing that you are searching for.

Yes, even accidents that cause illness are a result of wrong thinking, as well as diseases that you contract, even infection. If your body is truly in harmony with your mind, then your mind is in accord with what is natural, in harmony with the Universe. You will discover, at that point, that you will be immune to infection.

A strong will, strong mind, and a healthy body is an attitude that is important here. If you have an attitude that nothing can harm you as long as you take the proper steps to prevent it in every way, then you will have good health. You can learn about preventative measures from books and knowledge, but seek first the Spirit within, as it is necessary to know that it takes wisdom to act on this knowledge. *Have balance in life*. Be as the merged triangles, the six-pointed star, which is the symbolic meaning of balance in life, the center path of life. Be not a follower nor oppose others. Have your own path but be willing to have others follow you. You must seek peace with yourself in life. Seek inner harmony. Seek to avoid confrontation with those things that would cause harm to you physically and mentally.

Eliminate the stress, the tension, that causes the illness to have a foothold, that allows infection to have a foothold. Yes, you must do these things. You must eliminate your ideas of having your desires fulfilled instantly and grabbing things quickly without thought and reflection, things like quick love, quick wealth, quick notoriety or fame.

You seek quick answers. As I said before, you are traveling down the highway of life at too fast a speed. You must slow up. You must observe things more carefully and, in doing so, you will find the answers to your questions in life. You will find the treasures that you seek right there under your nose, so to speak.

IV

AIDS In Our Society

"AIDS is a cry for help and understanding by certain elements of your community in this country. It is a cry to bring about a greater understanding that loving awareness need not be exclusive, but can be inclusive of all. . . . there has been a polarity, a separation, a real challenge to be at home within the sexes. In other words, there is no understanding that men and women have both female and male qualities.

It is as if a demonstration has been called for on a level at which beings from all sexual persuasions on this planet could come together and say that it is all right to love each other."

1

The Homosexual Community

Choosing to be Gay and Why

Soli

My friends, why do you find illnesses coming to the Earth plane such as AIDS–acquired immune deficiency syndrome? What is the immune system? It is that part of the body that defends you from all attack, cleanses you from germs and viruses that would get in and attack the body. Now, if your main-line defense system is breaking down, what does it tell you?

It tells you that the body doesn't want to exist any longer. And why should the body not want to exist? Remember always, first comes the thought and then comes the reality. It is, my friends, because you have thoughts of self-destruction. You have thoughts of self-dislike and self-loathing.Why does this happen to the homosexual community?

Consider what is happening. First and foremost, as children there has been a tremendous pressure in society against being homosexual. The Judeo and Christian traditions, as in most societies, have beliefs that it is wrong, that it is sinful, that it is a crime against nature, all these wonderful expressions. Let us say at the outset that *there is no right or wrong*. There is no such thing as an absolute morality imposed by God. Morality is a belief system imposed by human beings on each other. *Beliefs*, again. You grow up in a society where these beliefs are programmed deep within your subconscious mind.

As children, even if you did not understand the terms, you sat and listened to your parents and friends talking at the dinner tables, or around the fireplace, and everything was recorded within your subconscious. *The feelings behind those words were recorded most strongly.* Children hear the communication of the parents' feelings far more than the communications of the words. A feeling of judgment, of loathing, of dislike is programmed in.

You have become homosexual because that was your choice, and if you have chosen a lifetime to be homosexual, you made that choice before coming here. You chose a somewhat difficult lifetime where you need to learn self-love in a very hard and harsh way. You know you will have those programmings as a child and as you grow up, you try to overcome them. There are many within the homosexual community who would say, "That doesn't bother me; what people think of me does not matter." To a large degree, some can live with that attitude.

But, for most, deep down, is that feeling that society is perhaps right after all. "What if they are right? What If?" All these "what if's." It is the tendency of the homosexual community to gather themselves into each other, to reject all who are outside, to close themselves off from anyone who might attack, from anyone who might bring those beliefs to the surface, so that they have to examine them again. In the process of closing off to the rest of society, you close off to yourselves, you close off to your fellow brothers and sisters, you shut down the communication channels, the heart chakra becomes closed.

Some communication is required, so what happens then? All the attention is placed within the lower physical chakra region. The predominant attitude within the homosexual community is that of physical beauty: "How attractive am I to others? How many partners, sexual partners can I have? The more sexual partners I have, the more it proves that I am truly beautiful in some way." The concentration is on the shape of the body, be it masculine or feminine. This same emphasis on the physical body is also true in the heterosexual community, this continual harping on the physical aspects, but it is much more prevalent and focused in the homosexual community.

Now, let us look again at some of the karmic backgrounds of this. Why would an individual choose to be homosexual in the first place? As a male in previous lives, perhaps you had a wife that left you, and left you very lonely, and you couldn't find anyone else. In the next lifetime you couldn't find any female at all. Lifetime after lifetime you found yourself feeling less and less attractive to females, feeling that there was something wrong, that you were simply not sexually attractive. So you say to yourself, "All right, this time I am going to go the other way; I am going to choose to have a lifetime where I deal with males." So you do. But you are still carrying that same idea. You have to prove yourself by proving that you are sexually attractive to another. The more sexual partners you have, the more sexually attractive you can prove yourself to be; the greater worth you have.

Why is it that AIDS seems to come to those who are most promiscuous? First and foremost, my friends, *there is nothing wrong with promiscuity*. From our perspective, sexual union is a communication, in a very high form, a very spiritual form. The more communication you have the better. It is not promiscuity that creates disease, any kind of sexual disease, it is *the thought form behind it.*

Those who go to the bathhouses are communicating that they want physical contact, quick physical union. They don't want to know the other people's names, they don't want them to know theirs; they don't want to open up, or let anyone know them. The self becomes quite locked up. It is physical only, in desperation only.

It is that thought form that allows that disease to take hold. It is a communication, again, from the Higher Self telling you, "Look, if you do not open your heart to others and to yourself, if you do not truly learn to love yourself and accept yourself and if you do not learn to truly go beyond those beliefs that have been placed there within your subconscious by society, then there is absolutely no point in staying on the Earth plane any longer." My friends, AIDS is but one form of leaving the Earth plane. There are many other ways, but you will find many within society who will be choosing to leave the Earth plane through that particular agency called AIDS.

81

Mirrors of Society

Dr. Peebles

You are all intensely aware of the homosexual society manifesting AIDS. AIDS is actively transferred and has been around for many generations, though undefined, through those who are *not* homosexual. I would say that already in your Western worlds, including the United States, AIDS was existing in many forms, in many people, before it was considered to be a sexual disease. *It is not a sexual disease.* Sexuality is certainly a way of transmitting it, but it is not a sexual disease. It is not a curse upon the homosexuals, and it is also not that homosexuals are doing a specific service to humanity. The illness was there. The illness is going to manifest with or without homosexuality.

The anxieties and the fears of the homosexuals have a more active impact on a physical contact level; the mucous membranes, the saliva, the blocks of emotions and beliefs. Combining these elements with their fears, their anxieties, many implanted by parents and society, makes them more susceptible. Do you understand? Your societies have implanted so much anger, guilt, and frustration in homosexual contacts that you have actually made them the vulnerable point.

I do not terribly approve of the term "victim." I am saying they are not victims of other attitudes, for they do not have to take those attitudes as their own. They become victims, if such a thing is possible, of their own willingness to become over-influenced, over-reactive to their own programming and training. Certainly, if you are looking for a common denominator, it is the lack of acceptance, the lack of growth, the lack of willingness to accept the homosexuals as human beings, growing in their own time, space, and way.

And so, if you are looking for a common denominator, it would be the negative programming of people who chose to be exactly what they are. Remember, my friends, that homosexuals *chose* that reality. It was not designed after they were born. It is the same for them as it is for the saint, the spiritual/religious leader, the prostitute, or the thief. They chose bodies long before they were born. They should be allowed the same.

Dong How Li

It is important for you to understand and to have some sense of an overview about homosexuality, since AIDS appears to be rampant in the gay community. If heterosexuality is the norm, so to speak, then homosexuality and bisexuality are the contraries. Now, what the contrary does is to provide a mirror. The mirror is designed to show the opposite, or the reflection, or a different perspective of what is the so-called "norm."

Now, I have a great question about what is the definition of norm, as it usually means statistical. What is different from the numbers, the norm, in this case, is homosexuality or bisexuality. That which is not part of the norm is, by nature, designed to reflect back to the majority that which the majority is *disowning,* what the majority is *not* doing. So, therefore, I am going to define norm as that which is normal and possible in nature. Homosexuality, bisexuality, and all the varieties of sexual expression are possible and indeed natural and normal, regardless of the statistics.

So, then, what is happening here has partly to do with the attempt to show so-called "straight" people what they have disowned within themselves. First and foremost, this applies to men, because they are the primary vehicle for AIDS now in this culture, to show men what they have disowned in their relationships with each other. Many straight men, to this day, do not wish to know about brotherhood, do not want to deal with affection between men from fear of it becoming sexual. The fear of it becoming sexual means they disown all of this whole way of being with each other. This denouncement, this renouncement, this repression, promotes violence, promotes competition, and even promotes a way of relating to women that is unfulfilling to both men and women.

Now, if the statistical norm–straight men–accepted this way of relating with each other, which is fuller and more balanced, the catch is, it need not necessarily be sexual. It might be occasionally sexual but it would not be rampant, and that is what the fear is. But the fear is unjustified. What makes homosexuality rampant is the initial repression that forces it outside of the self into something else.

The norm becomes fixated in heterosexuality, rather righteously, and the opposite, or that which is contrary, does the same. It becomes fixated in *its form of expression*. Neither one is truly appropriate. Both are truly stuck. Neither is capable of experiencing the *full range* of human love and its physical expression.

Now in the homosexual community you have a disease that is attacking the immune system. It is as if the homosexual community is saying, "We don't know what to fight, we don't know how to fight. We are open to invasion by something that is weak outside of the body, but inside of the body is most deadly."

The gay people are on the frontier, so to speak. They are outside the statistical norm. They are disrespected, rejected, and disowned. And it is the disowned aspect of the norm which places them on the frontier. This is true about any oppressed group. Because it is contrary and a mirror, it reflects back that which is diseased in the culture. In this culture, however, it is not respected because no one wants to own that which has been disowned.

The appearance of this disease, on this particular frontier, suggests what is already wrong in the male population in this culture. They do not know what they are fighting for anymore. They do not know how to love the softer aspects of their own maleness. Those secrets of being men are gone, lost. Straight men, like gay men, define masculinity for themselves, as well as others, by their penises. The rest of the male heart is unknown.

The appearance of AIDS in this culture is opening up the possibility for shedding light on the unknown portion of the male heart. Now, if you doubt what I am saying, just look at what is happening in the families of these gay men with AIDS. In most cases, it is forcing communication which was never possible before. It is forcing people to reconcile their differences in life-styles, values, and judgments.

The lessons inherent in the disease have first to do with knowing what to fight, when, how, and who. Second has to do with reconnecting and reestablishing communication between the part of the male heart that is known with the part that is unknown. The part that is

84

unknown has to do with brotherhood and cooperation between men. It does not necessarily need to be expressed sexually, although, as I have said before, occasionally in nature that occurs and it is all right. It is only another aspect of the human psyche.

Any oppressed group exaggerates what is already in the culture. For instance, those who criticize gay men for being promiscuous ignore the promiscuity among straight men where, in many cases, promiscuity is even honored. You see, that is the mechanism of disowning: "The problem is out there; therefore, I escape responsibility." That is obviously not true. One cannot escape that way because what is out there, *the mirror,* will push it back onto you. Those who are on the frontier get it first, but if the war is not fought on the frontier, it comes in behind the lines, does it not? Those on the frontier, in almost every other culture, are respected. That doesn't mean that you allow them to die for you. It means that you use what they are showing you to own within yourself.

Suppressing Emotions

Ting-Lao

Using the word suppress is very important because AIDS suppresses the auto-immune system. As you *suppress the emotions, you also suppress the auto-immune system.* For example, you hear an unkind remark and your emotions say, "This is not right. I should say something to that person who has said this prejudicial comment." But you suppress the response, the fighting back.

This virus has come into being first in the gay community because they cannot stand up for themselves and fight. They believe that society has put them into slots with certain ideas about them and there is nothing they can do to fight back. Deep inside they have this feeling, "This is how I am and society may think I am like this or that, but I cannot change society. So I will just live by myself." This is symbolic of not fighting back, of not fighting back in society and claiming one's self-hood. This allows society to continue to think these ill ideas. And it has ramifications in the auto-immune system.

85

What happens is that the auto-immune system turns against itself. The virus lives in the auto-immune system, in the T-cells. So if one increases the power and amount of the T-cells, this increases the power and amount of the virus. It is very confusing, and if you look at it symbolically, this confusion is in the gay community. There is confusion about who is friend and who is oppressor.

Being Non-Communitive

Soli

Why is it that most of the people within the homosexual community seem to be deciding to make their transition through the agency of AIDS? Please note our choice of words, *"Choosing* to make their transition through the agency of AIDS." Why does it seem that the majority making this change are the most promiscuous? Well, it is not simply because they are promiscuous, but it is the style of sex that they are having. Look at the impersonality of it, the physicalness of it, the lack of true contact with another individual, the isolation, the locking away of self. They are saying, "I really do not want to open myself up to anyone, and I will pretend that I am communicating through quick, physical sex."

And it is true, there is communication with quick physical sex. However, look at the thought form within that. Look at the belief which seems to be that by being who you are, you are not worthy of being upon the Earth plane. You do not wish to have others truly see who you really are.

Most of your difficulties, my friends, (and you are very well aware of this if you answer yourselves honestly) are with having *true communications* with each other and between each other.

The Polarity of Separateness

Dong How Li

You already know, medically, that the AIDS virus and cells appear in every living human being. Like cancer and other deadly diseases, the trigger that makes them multiply, explode, indeed, beyond repair, has to do with your values, your beliefs, your refusal to take stands and your refusal to own the parts of yourself that are important and powerful to you.

Zoosh

AIDS is a cry for help and understanding by certain elements of your community in this country. It is a cry to bring about a greater understanding that loving awareness need not be *exclusive,* but can be *inclusive.* On this planet, due to your religious and philosophical evolution of thought, there has been a polarity, a separation, a real challenge to be at home within both genders. In other words, there is no understanding that women have both female and male qualities, and that men have both male and female qualities. So, there is a basic separateness that has occurred between on a physical level.

On many other planets, there is the total understanding that to be of oneself, it is possible to incorporate masculine and feminine traits within one body. This occurs more on an emotional, mental, and soul-light level than on a physical level. AIDS is nothing more than a dramatic sense of drawing attention by a particularly responsible segment of your community on this Earth.

Realize that your *now* experience on this planet is one in which the *squeaky wheel gets the grease,* so to say. It takes a drama in order to draw attention to the idea that something is being overlooked. Many members of the gay community have gotten together at the soul or unconscious level to say, "Let us draw attention to the idea that love and loving has been very exclusive on this planet, up to now. Let us draw attention to the idea that it need not be so, that it can be much more inclusive, that it can be more simply a sharing of love between individuals who, in that moment, love each other." There need not be this great, almost apocalyptic disease idea.

It is as if a demonstration has been called for on a level at which beings from all sexual persuasions on this planet could come together and say that it is *all right* to love each other. It really comes down to this: if everyone would care to include in their thoughts and beliefs

87

that it is all right for people to love each other physically, mentally, emotionally, and spiritually as well, then it may not be necessary to have any disease.

If it takes a demonstration like this by a community that is willing to make sacrifices in order to make the point clear, then so be it. But for all of you, including members of that community, demonstrations could be made by simply stating that it is all right to love each other. It is all right to love each other. Simply that. Understand that it could, if repeated over and over, become watchwords of inclusivity instead of perpetuating the exclusivity that has gone on.

Lacking Self-Love

Soli

Have you noticed the number within your homosexual community who seem to have great self-destructive urges, who want to destroy themselves through drugs and alcohol, who cannot wait to get off this Earth plane, because they cannot bear to be here, and who do not like their lives?

Self-dislike and self-hate stems from past lives, my friends. Yet you have chosen to be a homosexual, you have chosen to be a part of this vibration. Why? So that you could learn love, love of self and love of others, a total unconditional acceptance of self. And that means, my friends, *not accepting society's belief systems about yourselves.*

Understand that the Judeo-Christian tradition runs strong and deep in this country and in many others. You have not escaped those belief systems. You have grown up with them. They have been implanted in your subconscious minds. However much you protest that they do not affect you, they do. However much you say that you like your life-style and who you are, those belief systems are still there. The subconscious is saying, "No, you don't really believe that at all. You are only pretending." And the subconscious mind and those beliefs are saying that what you are doing is actually a crime against nature. It is a sin; therefore, you will be punished by God. These judgments would have absolutely no effect unless you, your-

88

self, agree with them. Those beliefs are deep within your subconscious minds and deeply held fast.

They need to be found and brought into the light. They need to be changed, turned around, dealt with, blessed and released, but not fought with. You do not fight with the sub-conscious mind. You *bless and release* those thought forms that you find no longer of value to you in your life. Then you turn that belief system around and replace it with a different belief system, one that suits your life better, allows flowingness, freeness, and a projection of self.

My friends, there is no one way to behave upon the Earth plane. If we were to say that there is *one way,* then it would be that way which gives you the *greatest fulfillment* and feeling of *creativity within your life.* Dare to be different, dare to be outrageous. Dare to do those things that you feel *you* want to do and not because society says that you must do them, but because you truly feel that it is for your highest evolution. That is your best way forward for your own life.

2

The Heterosexual Community

Master Adalfo

People are believing that AIDS is only going to affect one segment of society. This is not so. Any people with the characteristics we speak of–fear, abuse, believing in lack, etc., need to look at their lives. They need to look at their belief systems. This gift of learning will help them solve their lives and make it less appropriate for them to develop AIDS.

It is true that the disease is spreading more widely in other circles. It has been, in fact, for some time in the heterosexual community, particularly with those who are drug abusers. This has not been publicized. At first it was just too convenient to say, "Oh, it's only *those people*." And many people thought it wouldn't affect anyone who was living a so-called "righteous life."

This goes along with the same idea that AIDS is a punishment from God. And if it is a punishment from God, it is only going to get those other people, not them. I want people to see that it can affect every single segment of society, and it is not dependent upon your sex life. For example, drug abusers, who risk it very heavily, are sharing needles, not bothering to have their own supply.

Remember that the whole idea of addiction is about abundance and lack. It is about seeing a world where there is no abundance and the only way to feel good is by using a substance. Those who are drug abusers are ignoring the risks they are taking, but of course, they choose to ignore *everything*. That is how addictive people are. They ignore much of the evidence because it only makes the world worse to them. Instead of doing anything about it, they say, "Oh well, I'll feel better when I have my shot, or I'll feel better when. . ." And they do, for a time. And when they begin to come down and see the world for how it is, then they have to have another shot because they don't want to see it.

Also, AIDS now is being transmitted by prostitutes and bisexuals. What this may do is create another shift and it may (though we hope it does not) push you all back to the prudish, Victorian sexual values. People are always seeking balance. After they become tired of being sexually repressed, they go the other way and become promiscuous, which is where we are now. And now, people are not really comfortable with that anymore. There is a possibility that they will go all the way back to being repressed again instead of finding a place in the middle that is comfortable.

This disease is making people start to look at their sex lives and at how comfortable or uncomfortable they are with their attitudes. They may be finding that the casual attitude of one night is not gratifying to them. This attitude is very similar to that of the homosexual who is not willing to delay instant gratification in lieu of companionship, nurturing love, and caring.

Soli

Why would a heterosexual get or "catch" a sexual disease? Imagine, my friends, a husband who is married, who goes out and has sexual relations with another female. He has probably already made up some lie, some excuse to his wife for going out. When he has sexual union with that other female, he is constantly in a state of guilt. If it continues for any length of time, he will always be totally worried that his wife is going to find out, and that he will lose what he has there. How can you have joy, true joy in the sexual union when all those thoughts are running through your mind? It is the *thoughts* that allow that disease to take hold. It is not the act in itself; it is the belief system behind it and the thought form behind it.

What is the way out of this? As with all things on the Earth plane, the way out is to learn to love the self, to truly accept who and what and where you are at this time, right now, exactly as you are, for that is *your choice*. That is what you are creating for yourself. That is what the Higher Self is experiencing. Love is a very misunderstood term. Love, from our perspective, is the total, *unconditional, non-judging acceptance of another's reality*. Love of self is an unconditional acceptance of yourself.

Women

Dong How Li

Women have a little easier time in this culture and, curiously, this disease is not affecting them in quite the same way. However, there are things for them to learn in this too. One of them has to do with allowing men to find their own softness according to the mysteries of being male. One of the things that is mistaken in this culture is that women feel that they can teach men how to be soft, how to be gentle. Not true. Only men can teach other men the mysteries of being men. Only women can teach other women the mysteries of being women. That is how it has always been. The rites of initiation are performed by members of the same sex who are older, wiser, and more experienced.

The lesson for women in this, then, is to allow men to do this exploration among themselves, indeed, to encourage them and be willing to step back and do the great feminine thing of making space and allowing. And in their relationships with men, women must come forward and relate, not by trying to be male in a business or a competitive way, but by trying to be a female and strong in womanliness. If this is done, there will be less competition between men and women. Each will understand the other. The man will understand that the woman cannot be strong in the way that he is and vice versa. The woman will understand that the man cannot be soft in the way that she is.

These are truly the mysteries. This is why this disease is so devastating, so powerful and frightening because *sex and death are mysteries.* One approaches the mysteries with respect. If one approaches them with fear, one is usually destroyed.

Children

Enid

If the being affected with AIDS is a child, then it's an experience that is needed to be felt throughout the entire family, perhaps by neighbors as well.

Outside of a very terrible war experience, there are very few experiences in which people feel quite so helpless. They see something happening and are not able to do anything about it. They experience this yearning kind of loving, "I wish it were myself instead of this darling child." They feel this great wanting to succor and take care of the child. It elicits all kinds of feelings.

Now, I wouldn't want, for a minute, to sound heartless because I understand the feeling that people have when these things are going on. When experiences are deep and rich, the rewards are also rich. The more dire an experience is, the heavier it is, the greater the reward.

So this might comfort those with children who are experiencing AIDS. Realize that your child has agreed to play a certain part in the family, to help the family grow in their expression of love and compassion in a way they would never grow without it. It's almost as if the child is saying, "I'm doing this for you. I'm helping you in your growth and in your loving."

The being himself who has agreed to such a terrible experience is exceedingly brave and must be treated as such. All beings are not willing to experience it. The experience of AIDS has to do with others observing the ones afflicted, observing their courage and reactions. If you'll notice, many who have AIDS speak with great courage and you find yourself very moved by that. You don't see them kicking, screaming, and feeling sorry for themselves. These are very brave individuals. Imagine what a brave individual a child is who is willing

93

to have such a very deep experience. This is one of the ways in which we measure our lives here, by the depth of our experiences and our willingness to experience them, and by the grace with which we come out of them.

Dr. Peebles

You may ask why children develop AIDS? Their souls *chose* to come into a body that would have a blood transfusion, that would have a transplant that was already affected by another gland or organ. They chose that body before they were born. As difficult as it is to observe, it is necessary to be as objective as possible, as empathetic as possible so that you allow the healing to take place on whatever level is best for the soul.

It's much easier to say, "Oh, that poor child. Oh, that poor person. They're not a homosexual. They must not deserve it." As I have stated previously, AIDS is not a sexual disease. It is a disease that is being transferred in so many other ways because it is not a curse, it is not a negative. AIDS is only another cleansing process.

Dong How Li

I don't think you can deprive children of their pain. That is part of being human and living. But you can share the wisdom of what we are presenting in this book, and know that you plant a seed by doing this. Both the child and the parent have chosen this. It is important that both the parent and the child begin to realize that they have done so. If any of you are helping such people (AIDS patients or their parents), part of your job is to remind them and to reconnect them to their original purpose, their original soul program and path. If you do that, then they can face this war as a hero.

You see, all of these people have *chosen* AIDS. Many of them, as you know, have forgotten why. They need to be reminded of that choice and helped to explore and find why so they can come with their full selves and confront this, and learn how to be a true warrior for themselves.

3

The Response Of The Church

Dong How Li

When religious leaders point fingers and claim that God is punishing, ask yourself, "Who do they feel is God?" They themselves are God. The people who have AIDS are God. *We are all God.* So who is God?

The part of God they know is punishing. The part of God others know is enlightening, is teaching. The part of God some AIDS patients are finding is a God of love and allowance.

There is no finger pointing from heaven and saying, "These people are evil." If there were a finger pointing from heaven saying who is evil, it would be pointed at those who *pass judgment* despite their very own religion and their very own Godhead, Jesus Christ. But, of course, they do not wish to look at this.

Remember that any sexual disease is called venereal. That means that it is a disease of love, named after the Goddess Venus. Does that make love evil? No. It means, however, that *how you love* needs to be looked at. So the finger here is saying, "Pay attention." It is not saying, "You are evil."

Zoosh

Understand that many of the religious and philosophical leaders have helped to bring about your current situation—although lovingly,

95

believing that they were doing what people wanted them to do. But, just like political leaders will not know what it is you want them to do until you make your opinions known to them, it is necessary for religious people to create somewhat of an outrageous statement, to really fly in the face of their religion. All religions sit on a base of love. If they do not sit on a base of love, they do not sit too long.

Condemnation flies in the face of the basic foundation of any religion. It is important for the world religious leaders to begin to know that their flocks do not wish to hear their fellow beings condemned. It is no longer necessary to create a lesser class so that people who are insecure have someone who is lower than they are.

So, understand that the issue is not whether you choose to be a homosexual. The issue is that some believe the idea of love (physically and emotionally) between people of the same sex is fundamentally wrong. Love between individuals of the same sex or opposite sexes cannot be wrong. *Love is love.* Is love wrong?

The issue is communication. How will we know, as a society, that there are polarized points of view if they do not come to the surface in a dramatic way? This is similar to not putting a stop sign on a corner until there have been a few accidents. You do not do something about a situation until it comes to the surface. This is the purpose of such apparent polarity.

Ting-Lao

There is not only vindictive behavior from some church leaders, but also anger of some people toward God and the church. They are saying, "Why has this happened to me? I have been a good and gentle person. I have never hurt anyone. I have lived my life well. Why is this happening to me?" Of course, this is the question surrounding any devastating illness. And again, it goes back to the need to be responsible and grow up and re-parent oneself and each other, and not to be looking for an outside source for enlightenment.

I do not have much comment about church leaders because it is quite obvious. They are being uncaring and unreligious, even though they often say they are religious. And hopefully they will learn. I

96

encourage you all to stand up and help them see what they are doing. Do not say, "Oh, that is what they are doing and I will just do my own thing." We need to help each other and help humanity grow together. Publicizing and speaking out is important, speaking to them in ways that will help them understand.

In some churches, there is much controversy about condom use. Why do our spiritual leaders continue to stand in the way of our progression? Why would they encourage people to be unconscious and careless, caring less about another and themselves? This is a major question for them to be asking themselves, because we do not feel that it is right to be talking out *against* precautions that can help people care for themselves and each other. We pray to the leaders of religion to begin working in all ways with the people, be willing to change and not perpetuate the same ideas and belief systems as before.

The issue of AIDS is causing waves in many religions as they struggle with the question of letting those with AIDS in the church or not, and with how much to help. It is good that AIDS has come to stir up these issues, and it is one of the good things that will come from this time, but I am not saying it was worth it. It is one of the things that will happen, but we wish it could have happened in an easier way, a more conscious way, instead of this punitive way.

Dr. Peebles

The comments about punishment and God's wrath are another wonderful opportunity for the churches to validate their belief systems, to validate many of their own psychological anxieties, to validate many of the programmings that were imposed upon them. It also is another way to scare people back into the church to build their coffers.

Master Adalfo

All religions, if taken to their highest level, are alike. You can see that. It is very clear. But people are not liking that similarity. They

97

always want to *see the differences*. They bring religion down to its lowest level and they see all those little factions, the tiniest little bits of difference. They concentrate on the differences, not on the similarities. They take away all the light by concentrating on them. The essence of the Christ is omitted. You talk to Southern Baptists and Northern Baptists. Do they talk about Christ? No, they argue about how they are different. You have arguments based on the big difference between Protestants and Catholics. They like to argue about the Virgin Mary. Nobody talks about the essence of her, who she is, the Mother of Christ.

You, here on this part of Earth, are thinking about how Christianity has been corrupted, but the same thing happens to all religions. You look at all the different divisions in Buddhism. There are many different factions and they are all talking about their little differences. The ecumenical spirit should be that everyone concentrates on what is the same.

You can send light to those in the churches who are working in a positive and loving way. You can also send light to those who are not because if they don't have any light, they certainly need it. And that includes those misguided souls who are saying that AIDS is a punishment from God. They need even more light because they have none. They have so little light they don't even know *what* God is. They have a great belief in a punishing God. Why do you suppose they enjoy living in a Universe where God is always punishing? Does it make them right? Yes, and that is why they like it; they get to be right. God is not punishing them because they are right. And if they don't have the disease, then God isn't getting them. Wait until someone with those beliefs gets AIDS.

V

The Many Reasons For AIDS

"Fear brings you that which you fear. It manifests circumstances that allow you to have first-hand experience of what it is that you fear, so that you can get over it and move beyond it. . . .Fear brings so-called fearful situations to you so that you can discover this fact, it creates your reality and circumstances. The mere fact that you fear AIDS means that you are actually saying to yourself that you can catch it."

1

Physical, Emotional, Mental
And
Spiritual Aspects

Ting-Lao

There are physical, emotional, mental, and spiritual reasons about why some people come down with this illness and why others do not. First, let us look at the situation from a physical point of view. Physically, it has to do with general health care. For example, general cleanliness with intravenous drug users is an obvious problem. Unsafe sexual practices are also an obvious problem. People can get exposed to the virus more than one time and this makes a physical difference. Having promiscuous sex does add to the physical aspect of risk because people can be exposed to different strains of the virus and bring more stress on the system and, thus, are more likely to come down with the disease.

Oftentimes people do not care for themselves very well. They do not eat well or exercise enough, which are the known basic ways to care for one's body. The immune system, the lymphatic system, is what is necessary to address here. The ingestion of toxic foods and many antibiotics throughout life creates an overload in the lymphatic system. The frequency of illnesses in childhood and early adulthood can also weaken the auto-immune system. So, these are physical aspects that can affect people, whether they manifest these problems or not because the virus is the same in all bodies.

There is a metaphysical aspect here that crosses over into the emotional, and that is fear. Fear is the food of this disease. So, people

101

who are afraid that they will get it, or will die from it, are creating food for the disease. In a metaphysical sense, this fear affects whether some people will come down with the disease or not. Fear is a big factor.

The reason that this disease has entered the American society through the gay male community is primarily because of the symbolic relationship of the auto-immune system with the rest of the body, as they both are always having to fight for their way. It is a metaphysical relationship and these people need to fight for their rights to be as they wish. Because their energy systems are always on the defense, they get worn out. This also has ramifications in the physical defense systems—the auto-immune system—causing it to become weak. The auto-immune system should sometimes have to fight and sometimes rest; however, it is always on alert, because the energy systems are always on alert.

This is another emotional reason why some people are more prone to come down with this condition. It involves those who are fighting more on a mental level than on an emotional level. They are fighting with the words and thought forms of other people around them. In most cases it is an internal battle and is not fought outwardly. They are getting attacked, subtly, usually by little comments, little subtle innuendos throughout society, throughout television, throughout the press. They do not have the opportunity to fight directly. This is a good point because they are fighting on mental levels and feeling like they have to have their defenses up because they are always being attacked, but not able to have an actual battle.

The physical defense system, then, breaks down as a result. There arises a weakening of the will because of this constant bludgeoning from society. Now this, of course, has to do with the gay community particularly because they often come from backgrounds where they were abused mentally, emotionally, or physically. So, again, they were being attacked and were not having the chance to fight back. The other person was too strong, too powerful.

Mental reasons have also to do with the fear—the mental fear, not only the emotional fear—of having this thought form or this idea around them that expresses, "Oh, they are going to get AIDS and

102

therefore die." The metaphysical laws which state that thoughts are actual things are stating the truth, but it is not the *only* truth, just part of it. When one thinks a thought over and over again, it can affect the energy around him. So, when people start worrying about whether they have AIDS or whether they are going to get it, this actually attracts it to them. The thought forms and the thought ideas, which are going through the mind field surrounding that particular person, links the fear with that which is feared. Your mind field becomes magnetic through any strong idea that is held within it and draws that situation which best matches that particular strong idea to itself. So, in that sense, worrying about it does make a difference. Worrying also affects the nervous system through the physical stress one creates as a result. This is another mental aspect of attracting disease. That part of the heterosexual community who have AIDS are more mental and their karmic lessons, their karmic teachings to the culture are more mental.

The spiritual is the most complicated aspect, as this often involves people who had no thought that they might get it. It also involves the children who contact it through blood transfusions. Often they are serving a spiritual purpose by getting it, by participating in this whole section of society that is experiencing the AIDS disaster. They have chosen to participate in that way, not on a conscious level, of course, but on the soul level because there is much for humanity to learn through this disaster about caring for each other and caring for oneself, about equality and bigotry, and medically, about viruses. Spiritually, it is sometimes a person's way to pass on into progression, into the soul's progression. Some people choose cancer, AIDS, car accidents; there are many ways. When it is time for the soul to decide, then, sometimes that happens. This is the spiritual aspect.

We are not saying that it happens in all cases. Sometimes, as we have said, it is physically based, sometimes emotionally based and sometimes it is more mentally based. Each person is different and each strain of the virus is different. For example, in the gay community, because AIDS is often transmitted in the very creative act of sexual union, those who develop the virus are indeed teachers of physical karma. They have karmically come to learn in this manner, and then they, in turn, teach the culture what they have learned. So it is that each individual will decide what he is to learn as he copes with the disease. The people around him who are exposed to the phenomenon of this epidemic will receive lessons in turn.

The intravenous drug users are using drugs mainly because of emotional imbalances. This is the emotional learning and teaching group. They are learning from the disease in the emotional sense, and they are teaching the culture in an emotional sense, focusing on energy interaction.

The other people, the children and others from the three groups that I have mentioned, come to the Spiritual Teacher groups to learn, as well as to advise. People who always question and wonder about the meaning of death and disease are learning about these different aspects and then, in turn, are teaching the culture about them. This is why different groups of people are being exposed to AIDS and accepting the disease.

There are certain things that we could say, but will not because experience seems to be the best teacher for every individual. The culture must be stirred up enough by this energy so that it can decide how it thinks and feels about these different aspects on its own.

2

Fear,
The Food Of AIDS

What is Fear?

Kyros

All negative illusions which you perceive are based on fear. Christ was always saying, "Fear not!" Why? Because He knew fear would bind you and imprison you and prevent you from experiencing a full and abundant life. He also knew that fear of anything is ego-based and the ego's main function, as you know, is to maintain and protect the physical vehicle. The ego knows that once the Spirit is released from the vehicle, it no longer has either purpose or power.

Ting-Lao

Fear is a condition of low energy, low vibration. Having that constriction of energy molecules in the body is like a chemical substance in the body. So, as you raise the personal vibration through knowing self and loving self and others, it raises that vibration so that fear cannot live in the body. Fear vibrates at one level, and when the body is vibrating with health, fear falls apart because it cannot vibrate at the level of a healthy body.

Many people call fear a thought form, but we want to give it more of a concrete chemical structure than just a thought form because lots of people think lightly of thought forms. They don't realize that thought forms are very powerful and they are very real. So, think of fear as being free-floating anxiety, as if it were an entity itself.

How Fear Attracts That Which Is Feared

Soli

Fear brings you *that which you fear*. It makes manifest circumstances that allow you to have first-hand experience of that which you fear so you can get over it and get beyond it. The subconscious mind fears what it does not know. Once it has experienced something it feared, it realizes that the experiences were far less onerous than the fear of the event.

Your fear, in itself, creates your reality, creates your circumstances. The mere fact that you have fear means you are saying to yourself, "I can catch this."

So, if you have fear of something, my friends, what does that mean? It means that within your mind you are saying, "I have the potential of experiencing this very negative thing." You are programming yourself to have the experience. If you have never heard of a disease, oftentimes you will not catch it, unless there is the need for the experience. You do not *catch* disease. You make yourself *susceptible* to it by your thoughts and your needs.

Dr. Peebles

My friends, you transmit germs to every being that crosses your path. For instance, you have a cold. Your cold is in the room and everyone who comes in is exposed to it. They decided to enter the room. You didn't go out on the street and drag them in, did you? Some might say, "Oh, I hope I don't get it, I hope I don't get it." They've already got it. The ones who are saying, "Oh well, that's interesting. I hope she'll have a good time with it, hope it doesn't interfere too much with her productivity, hope one day it's no longer around her," they're not going to bother getting it.

Don't worry about what germs you may put out with your cold.

106

They're automatically going out anyway. Those acting in fear, they're going to get it anyway. If they don't catch it from you, they're going to be walking down the streets saying, "Oh, I hope I don't walk through any negativity. I hope I don't walk through any cold bugs." They're going to catch all of them from wherever they are.

So go into your stores, go into your offices. Do everything that you feel up to. When you have an illness, when you have a cold, when you have a headache, go out and do everything that you feel comfortable in doing.

But if you feel, "Everybody there might get sick," remember that *everyone there* is going to get sick only according to their willingness, their ability to call upon, to magnetize, to process it. It's all out there anyway. Everyone is going to be exposed to it. Let them discover what they're going to do with it.

Who are you to say, "Oh, but I should lock myself in my house. That way nobody will be exposed." I have a big surprise for you. All of your little cold germs, they don't understand wood and glass. They'll go out visiting anyway. Go into a laboratory and see how they have all kinds of things to try to make sure that the germs don't get out. They have all kinds of cleansing processes. They cleanse their scientists, they cleanse room by room by room to clear out all the germs because they don't know those viruses are not confined by time, by space, by steel, by glass.

The Fear of Lack

Master Adalfo

You might say that AIDS is a disease of fear. It is a second chakra disease: one of emotion—fear. And it is fear of not having enough, not having it when you want it. It is the feeling of, "If I don't take it now, there will not be any." It is wanting approval at any cost. It is much like going to McDonald's for quick fast food. It is wanting everything instantly, everything fast.

Now, if you are wanting a relationship, the more specific you can get in your list of qualities and traits, the easier it is for you to make

107

space in your auric field for the Universe to provide that to you. If you never take the time to do that, then you are always grabbing at whoever happens to walk by.

The measure of appropriateness of this is asking what is appropriate for you. But you must take the time to think that out first and then to make time for relationships to develop. Relationships do not develop in five minutes. So, you need to know clearly, in your mind, what qualities you want to feel with your emotions. You need to know about those things that you want in another person. Then be looking for those in people you meet. If you meet someone that seems to have some of those qualities, take time to get to know them, to understand them, to ask yourself, "Is this person really someone I would like to be with?"

This means believing in the abundance of the Universe and knowing that you don't have to have something *right this minute*. You can wait because it will be there for you. Obviously I do not mean there is only one person on the whole planet that is right for you. That is ludicrous. There are many. But if you do not know the qualities that you want, how will you know when one of those people is there?

Of course, if your culture did not have the great sexual repression that you have, then children would be freer to experiment sexually when they are younger. This is normal. But no one allows that, or *hopes* they are not allowing it (much goes on no one knows about). If that experimentation were allowed to go on as normal, people would have less *lack* feelings and they would also know more about what they want. But because they are so repressed, some people do not know what they want until they are in their twenties. So they are experimenting at that age instead of when they are seven or eight. So the child in them is not grown up at all. As adults, you must take charge of *that* little child. You must understand that you have a little rebellious child and how can you help them grow up? You do not want to be this little child forever.

There is nothing wrong with sexual attraction. The point is you do not decide on a relationship based *only* on that. You will be attracted to many people. You know you have body hormones which respond to them, it has little to do with anything else. This doesn't mean you want to be with that person. Your body might want to be with that person, but not you. The intrinsic *you* is not your body.

This disease does force those who are in danger of getting the disease (particularly homosexuals) to draw back and to take time in selecting a partner, taking time to evaluate. It is a letting go of childish things, of childish behavior, of saying, "This is my toy and I want it now!" It is letting go of old things, being open to new ones, being open to the essence of being an adult, a mature person. It is more an issue of maturity than just about *being* an adult. Presumably the two should go together, but that does not always happen.

Disease oftentimes can be seen as a process that gives you permission to draw back, to go to bed, to take time, to evaluate what is going on in your life. The same is true of AIDS. Often with this disease, those who are experiencing it have never taken the time to evaluate relationships in this way before. Never! It is really not an issue about homosexuality itself. This is not the key issue. It is about lack and abundance and waiting and taking time.

3

Immune System Breakdowns

The War Inside

Jesus of the Light

The AIDS experience is one of disassociation or re-establishment of the human race on this Earth. Your experience, albeit difficult and trying to those who directly experience it and to those who are exposed to those who are experiencing it, is merely a choice to redefine the impact of the human race on this planet. Some time ago, it was predicted that the idea of an Armageddon, or a war to end all wars, would take place on this planet. That idea has been replaced through time and experience with the idea of an *internal* Armageddon to be faced by all individuals on their own.

The planet that you live upon, Mother Earth, has chosen not to participate again in a war to end all wars, but Mother Earth is encouraging you all to experience that war within, so that you may know what war is really all about and to realize the many advantages of feeling peaceful, thinking peaceful, acting peaceful, and being peaceful.

The mistaken notion in the past, that war is the absence of peace, is not its total definition. War, in many senses, is the absence of freedom, the absence of joy and the absence of equilibrium. In that sense, it is now time to re-establish your own equilibrium on this planet. Equilibrium, in this sense, means balance; balance in

110

thought, in deed, and in action.

Understand that this experience of AIDS is a precursor to the idea of your experience of the internal Armageddon. AIDS is, as you perceive it, a disease associated with the immune system in your physical bodies. Your immune system, however, is primarily an attachment to the idea that disease is an enemy and that you do battle with disease so that a victor can be declared one way or the other. Understand that it is, in many senses then, equivalent to war. In order to have an immune system, you must need to feel a threat, a presence about you that owes its allegiance to something outside of yourself. Therefore, the idea of Armageddon, as applied to yourself now, is an influence which is not directed by yourself. It reaches out beyond your sense of control, beyond your sense of the ability to defend yourself and states that, "I am not able to protect myself in all situations."

The purpose of your internal Armageddon, then, is to help you to realize your own power to re-create and re-establish your reality as you experience it here on this planet. War, as you have experienced it in the past, does not create the idea of re-establishing your own internal identity through any means other than as a *winner* and a *loser*. This means that at least some of the people will have the ability to create their own reality denied them as the loser. Also, some of the people will have the ability to create their own reality beyond the ordinary responsibility to the self by dictating a reality for the losers, as the winners might do.

It is time to redefine the need for a physical immune system to address the idea that "I can be safe in my physical body on the Earth now, in its most loving and supportive sense." You need to acquaint yourself with a true sense of loving purpose in your lives. But for now, I must suggest to you that this loving purpose has not been served by the experience of disease and war. In that sense, you have developed over the years the need to protect and defend and, in some cases, attack in order to believe that you are defending something worthwhile in yourself.

The immune system is merely a physical manifestation of that very attitude within your physical body. The disease of AIDS and

111

other diseases which cause a breakdown in the immune system will gently or not so gently remind you of certain things: of the need to begin to establish within yourself a system of beliefs in your mind, a system of feelings in your emotions, a system of sensations in your physical body in order to guide you toward the internalization of the inspiration of your Spirit or your Soul Self as an active portion of your mind, your emotions and your body. The Soul or Spirit does not experience disease, it does not experience war. It does not need to experience an immune system or that which is a defender.

So, recognize that for you all to be truly happy now, to be truly fulfilled, it is necessary to recognize that the experience of AIDS is designed to draw your attention to the immune system. It is not to redefine the immune system as an enemy. It is rather to begin to replace it with positive thoughts.

Zoosh

All kinds of immune syndrome deficiencies will be classified under the broad heading of AIDS these days, because AIDS as a symptomology has been defined and categorized; therefore, making it possible to say that variations of the symptomology will fall broadly under the heading of AIDS. Understand that this worldwide phenomenon is something that is symbolic of the idea that an immune system is needed. It reflects the obvious thought of: well, you must need immune systems because you are not safe. There is danger. There must be a system to combat the danger from without.

Understand then that the primary emotion at the base of the need for any immune system is the fact that people do not believe that they create their own safety; so, in that sense, any immune system experience, as well as any disease at all, will be caused by primarily a lack of belief in personal safety.

The way to really approach this thought these days is, rather, to look at the idea, "What can I do to increase my own awareness of whether I feel safe?" It is time to take into consideration how comfortable you feel, how easy your day-to-day life is. This does not mean how easy it is in the sense of how your life might be accommo-

112

dated to fit into the pattern of total relaxation, but, rather, how easy it is in the sense of what you do to create comfort for yourself. Do you resist that which comes to assist you? Do you make combat with your friends and co-workers? Understand that it is important for you to create ease within yourself, to find comfort, not to submit to discomfort. In that sense, it is a time on your planet when people will be seeking to find comfort without feeling put upon and without creating a sense of anxiety for themselves.

I encourage you all out there, if you are in somewhat uncomfortable surroundings, either begin to treat yourself with more comfort and kindness within your surroundings or consider altering those surroundings.

4

Guilt

Soli

Again, it is not the sexual act in itself that creates the problem, it is the beliefs around it. When all of your teenagers grow up and start having sexual experiences and they have been taught to believe that it's bad and that it's wrong, this creates a tremendous pressure within the mind, creates tremendous self-disgust, self- hate.

You are seeing it in the homosexual community, but it is also endemic throughout the whole of your society. You are given this biological force, something absolutely wonderful, a *delightful expression of love* from one to another. Then you hedge around it with so much fear, with morality, with guilt, that you make it almost impossible to enjoy it. Still, it is something so powerful that you cannot ignore it. All you are doing is creating a society of guilty individuals and, of course, this is exactly what those in power want. Those who would dominate you with their religious beliefs, or their political beliefs, those who would maintain control of the population in any way, shape or form—for them, the best way to control is through guilt.

Give individuals something so powerful that they cannot leave it alone (it is seemingly like an addiction) and then make it into something that is a crime against nature, or a crime against God, for which you are going to be punished and go to hell for eternity! Think what *guilt you are placing in the mind of every individual.* At the same time you have set certain individuals or religions up as the only way out of their guilt, the only way to God. What tremendous power you are giving away. And that is why it is set up in this way. These moral beliefs are beliefs of control, of maintaining power for those individuals who would promulgate them. Those who would give away their power are those who do not want to take responsibility for their lives; they want to be controlled by these beliefs. And since they are controlled by those beliefs, they don't want to see anybody else in the society around them have personal freedom; so, they too try to control others around as well and spread the message, as it were.

We are totally for *increased education, increased understanding* of what this urge is, how to use it, and that sex *per se* does not create disease. Venereal diseases are transmitted through the guilt and the self-punishment within you because you feel guilty that you are creating that sexual act. It is what you believe about yourself and what you draw to yourself that creates the disease. It is not the mechanical act in and of itself. It is the motivation and the belief that always creates the illness, not the mechanics. We cannot stress that too highly.

Oppression

Dong How Li

There is AIDS in Africa, there has been AIDS in Europe where it is primarily homosexual. In Africa, the Caribbean, and in South America, AIDS affects the heterosexuals.

Again, the issue is invasion and the difficulties of knowing what to fight. All of these people who have this disease share a common denominator which is *repression;* they are all oppressed, whether that is due to sexual preference, race, economics, or religion.

When you are oppressed and turn the war on yourself, often you do so because you don't know where else to fight because the enemy is unseen. In sexual preference, in this country, that is very true. The laws are beginning to give more freedom to this issue, but the unspoken values are still a prison. This is also true in third-world

115

countries where dark peoples know there is prejudice against them, yet do not know where to fight because it does not confront them directly. They have no external thing to focus on. So it focuses inside and eats them from every direction. Part of what you want to do in the healing process is to help people find an *outside* focus to fight. That directs the energy, keeps it from generalizing and spreading all over the inside of the body.

5

Your Need
For
Experience

Enid

AIDS is an experience to remind us that this is a finite world. And at the same time you learn that this is a finite world, you're learning about your own infinity because these beings are dying. They are falling over like flies. They are just dying here and there and yet all the people associated with them are beginning to get closer to their own infinity. In that sense, it reminds us of both ends of that spectrum, that spectrum of the finiteness of the world and the infinity of beingness. Even this world is finite because we don't intend it to last forever. There's a lot of forever and this is just a spark of forever.

I think we can overblow this whole sense of what the meaning of AIDS is. If we could step back a little bit, we could see it as an experience, just as falling from a mountain and breaking one's leg is an experience. It is not a greater experience nor is it a deeper experience than many other experiences. For instance, consider the mother whose son has been lost in a foreign war, and who doesn't know for sure whether he's dead or incarcerated somewhere. That mother's experience is just as deep or deeper than having AIDS.

There are so many ways that we experience all these deep experiences. And the experience of mystery and wonder has really been enlivened because of AIDS. We put a man on the moon, we took close-up pictures of Mars, and yet here is this incredible disease that we don't seem to be able to do anything about. That is because people are

117

looking in the wrong direction. The right direction is from the Spirit.

If you tell someone who has AIDS that he decided to have the experience, he'll probably hit you in the snoot. He'll say, "I certainly didn't want this." Well, in his awake state, he didn't. If we chose everything from our awake state, our lives would really be totally different; but we don't. We are interacting with our reasons for being here. We are interacting with our own goals of what we expected our life experience to be, and it is very important that these things be fulfilled. The surprise is how they are to be fulfilled. Well, they're going to be fulfilled this way or that way or the other way, but they will be fulfilled.

For one, it's AIDS and for another it may be falling from a ship into the sea and staying there for three days before being rescued. It can be any manner of ways. It can be being lost in a cave for a week and trying to get out. There can be all kinds of ways in which the end product is achieved. Know that everything that you're reaching for is a part of your process. *Everything that you experience is a part of your process.*

The Evolution Of Growth

Dr. Peebles

There is no major cure found for AIDS at this point because it is a soul experience, individually and collectively. It is a natural evolutionary process and so it will not be cured before it has gone about its natural cycle and done what it was designed to accomplish. So often the human mind says, "Oh well, this is a terrible thing. We're going to find a cure." Rather than turning it over to the encouragement to live up to your soul's choices, you try to cure something that is incurable, that is a part of the natural evolutionary process. AIDS is not, then, something to fear. AIDS is something to recognize as little more than another opportunity for souls to be fulfilled.

It is no more negative than the wars that have been, and the wars that will be. And you all look back on all of the great plagues, and on the great wars and say, "Aha, but they were the elements that led us

118

to evolutional consciousness." The same will be true, in retrospect, of AIDS.

My friends, AIDS is here and now. How do we deal with it now? If we want to deal with it, don't be afraid. Don't say, "Oh, my goodness, I must escape!" If you came in to have it, you will have it whether or not you live in a cave for the rest of your life or whether or not you go out and carry on with every living human being, male, female, or otherwise. It is an attitude, and it is an attitude that must relate to your soul.

Ting- Lao

This virus, as well as any disease, is like a big kick in the rear end, telling you that something needs to happen now in the consciousness of this person and in the culture. Again, the person is a reflection of the culture and serves in this way to awaken the culture, to awaken their consciousness to greater possibilities. This is what it is: awakening the consciousness of people to what more is possible in life, and in themselves. I realize this sounds simplistic, trying to understand when life is not understandable. And you can make it work in many ways as you progress to understanding.

Taulmus

This sickness is now at epidemic proportions upon your land and is a signal for a cleansing. It is a time to set your houses in order, so to speak. Each of you, and your planet as well, whether conscious of the fact or not, is going through much change and upheaval which is triggering a time of renewal for all creation on all levels of physical and non-physical life.

As many of you know, new energies have been released upon your plane that are facilitating this time of transformation. Many of your space brothers, such as myself, and those souls who work from inner dimensions and more rarefied levels of thought, are stirring up the

119

light on your world. With this influx of high frequency energy on your plane, it would seem that many lives are falling apart, when, in truth, they can be seen as *falling together*. It often takes grist for the mill in order for it to run at its peak efficiency.

VI

Healing

"Healing, my friends, is facilitating an individual to heal themselves; to view their lives in a different way, to see what changes they need to make in order to assist them in the process of self-discovery. Everything is a process of learning to love yourself, to accept yourself exactly as you are. . . . Unless you open yourself and listen to communication from your Higher Self, it is forced to use the lower vibrations which you cannot ignore. You cannot ignore a physical illness, disability or so-called accident. You have to take notice. You have to discover what it is that the Higher Self is communicating. . . . Once you have seen those and dealt with them, healing is instant, absolutely instant."

1

All Healing
Is
Self-Healing

Soli

Healing implies that there is something wrong, that there is something that needs correction, that there is something within the physical body or the emotional body that is out of balance.

How do you heal? You must first understand what disease is. You understand that it is a communication from the Higher Self, physical, emotional or mental. You understand that you cannot truly eliminate disease from the Earth plane. You cannot eliminate disease from an individual life until that individual *understands* the communication. When your path upon the Earth plane diverges from that which you chose before coming here, you, as your Higher Self (for you are your Higher Self, not your physical body) communicates to you, provokes you, motivates you into change and, perhaps, into accepting change upon the Earth plane, within your life.

Disease is that communication. There is no need for it apart from that. There is no objective illness, no objective beliefs outside of what *you create for yourself*. There is no way that you can be a victim of disease or illness. You have disease or illness in your life out of *your own need,* your own need for change. There is no pain or suffering in any objective sense. Pain and suffering are always within the subconscious mind because of its resistance to change within your life.

There is some "thing" that comes forward within your life that you feel that you should do; your subconscious mind resists, tells you all the things that would go wrong if you moved on that path, and brings forward all the fears, all the doubts. That is the cause of pain and suffering. It is when the course of action that you know and truly feel you should take is not matched by your belief systems, when your beliefs tell you that if you follow that course of action you are in danger or in trouble. That is the cause of disease.

How then to heal? Obviously, the way to heal is to understand that communication and to take action. That is not always as straightforward as it might appear, of course. Otherwise there would be no disease on the Earth plane. Everybody would automatically heal themselves. *There are no incurable illnesses, only incurable people.*

It is the person that must heal himself. There is no such thing as a "healer." All beings have healing ability. You as healers cannot heal another individual without the permission of the individual's Higher Self. It is only at their request that you can heal. You can apply your arts to individuals and yet they will stubbornly refuse to be healed. Why? It is because the Higher Self *must communicate.* If they do not hear that communication, if they do not take action upon it, then there is *nothing* at all of any kind that will heal them. Nothing. No energy transference, no mechanical drug systems, nothing will heal them, for that communication must be followed.

Of course, once you have opened the channel by communicating, then communication will come through on that vibration. We are not saying that the Higher Self cannot communicate in that way; it is simply that it cannot initiate the communication. It tries extremely hard, but unless you open yourself and listen to that communication, you do not receive it. Therefore, the Higher Self is forced to use the lower vibrations which you cannot ignore. You cannot ignore a physical illness, disability, or so-called accident. You have to take notice. You have to discover what it is that the Higher Self is communicating. What is it within your life that you are not doing? What are you not perceiving? What are you not changing? What are you holding onto so dearly within your life that you will not let go? What belief systems do you have about yourself and your life that you cannot change or let go of?

124

Once you have seen those and dealt with them, healing is instant, absolutely instant. There is no need for the communication to maintain any longer. You can be cured instantly once you have understood and taken action upon that communication.

Now, there are times when there is partial understanding, when you understand partly what the communication is, and you begin to work upon it. You begin to change your life in some ways, but not in all. Then you can very often enlist the aid of others around you to assist, to help you balance the body in some ways with energy, with other forms of healing, with herbs, with nutrition, there are many other ways. This allows you to correct some of the minor imbalances so that you can deal more readily with the changes that you are making within your life. It is in effect, a rebalancing.

So, healing, my friends, is not healing at all. It is facilitating an individual to *heal themselves,* to view their life in a different way, to see what changes they need to make in order to assist them in the process of self-discovery. Everything is a process of self-discovery. Everything is a process of learning to love the self, to accept yourself exactly as you are. You do this by discovering and understanding who you are, learning to love that and then knowing that you can change and accept the change that comes forward in your life. However, you do not have to change if you accept where and what you are at any given moment.

Accept means total acceptance, without judgment, of where you are and what you are doing. As you accept everything that comes toward you, every aspect of life, do not allow the subconscious mind and its fears and doubts to stop you from taking that course of action.

You have no need for physical changes, you do not need to age. The body ages because of its resistance to change, just like any other disease. It does not have to be that way, and yet it is an important process, for the body weakens and finally gets to the point where the Higher Self can no longer sustain life within it because the individual needs to leave the Earth plane. Those people have not reached the stage where they can leave voluntarily (at will) and must find a way to leave the Earth plane. You cannot live forever. The Higher Self has not the slightest interest in living forever within one physical body.

125

The Higher Self hasn't the slightest desire to stay within one physical projection forever upon the Earth plane. It decides when there is no further growth to be had within that particular physical vehicle. The Higher Self decides when that physical vehicle should decay and end its present projection. And no healer upon the Earth plane will ever stop that from happening if the Higher Self does not feel that there is any future growth to be had.

Kyros

All illness and disease exists because you believe in illness and disease. Why do you believe in it? Because you have been programmed since your entrance (your birth) to believe in it. Since man's entrance on the planet Earth, he has believed in it. Look at your television advertising. From it, you surely must believe that in order to be human you must have the flu, headaches, backaches, stomach aches, arthritis, and so forth. Some even believe that they are destined for heart disease, cancer, diabetes, AIDS, herpes, and on and on. With all the programming, I am sometimes surprised that man has survived as well as he has.

On the other side of the coin, the programming which causes man to continue his belief in illness and disease also causes him to believe in healing. Does aspirin really make a headache go away, or is it your belief that aspirin will release you from pain and make it go away? This is something, perhaps, that you will never be able to scientifically prove, but I will tell you that if you did not believe that aspirin would help, it would have no effect. Your belief system is critically important in the bringing on of the manifestations of both illness and healing. If you have an illness and you do not believe in healing, self-healing is impossible.

All healing is self-healing, whether you ingest medications, undergo surgery, spend time with physicians, or offer yourself to any of the treatments within your current medical technology. To be healed you must believe in healing, you must trust that you can be healed and you must have faith in whatever method you have selected to trigger your own healing energies into action.

126

Self-healing begins first in your *belief in healing*. Healing is the manifested thought which erases the manifested thought of illness and disease. It involves reprogramming, and always when one desires to change how he thinks about something, there must be both the will and the willingness to do so. Healing has to begin in your own consciousness, since most illness can be traced back to negative ego vibrations and thoughts such as fear, anger, hate, resentment, guilt and so on. These must be dealt with. It is here that the real healing occurs.

What I'm trying to say is that an entity might have a properly functioning form which is seemingly free of disease and still be diseased if he harbors negative ego thoughts and vibrations. Another entity, on the other hand, may have what appears to be a diseased form and yet may not harbor negative ego vibrations and thoughts. Where it really counts, he is the one who is healed and healthy.

2

Physical, Emotional, Mental
And
Spiritual Aspects

Ting-Lao

If one has AIDS, there are physical, mental, emotional, and spiritual ways in which to deal with the situation. Physically, of course, you should be under a doctor's care. Look around for sensitive doctors who have cared for this condition previously. There is some insensitive physical care that is being given by some doctors who do not care about the person because he is gay, and similar situations like that. There are some doctors who are experimenting with drugs hoping to find a cure for AIDS. So, it is a good idea to look around and find a good doctor. Know that each day there are new medical advances in the area and do not give up hope. A medical breakthrough may come the next day, and there will be a cure for this disease.

Physically, one should also try to take the best possible care of oneself. Ask for help in caring for oneself because it is possible to live with AIDS after being sick from its effects and from its secondary infections. It is possible to conquer it. Life-styles must change. Responsibility issues must come out and be resolved. Anger and the fear that this virus eats or grows on must be addressed.

Moving to the emotional, sometimes psychotherapy can help one to deal with the problem. Many AIDS support groups deal with the problem of having AIDS. What we want to deal with is the problem of *life* and the interaction with life that has led to the opportunity of

128

AIDS getting into the body. Then fight that and stop it and change it to be strong. Fight for yourself in a way that many people have not been able to do; therefore causing the auto-immune system to give up. It is possible to conquer it and live with these viruses in your body.

There must be support emotionally, of course, you need someone to talk to and someone who will listen to you. Also, there needs to be direct psychotherapy, and if not, then there needs to be someone who loves you unconditionally and also conditionally in order to help you change and face matters. You see, we are taking the stance that AIDS is *a warning* that you need to change, not a death pronouncement. It is only a warning that you need to change, to take a hard look at yourself and decide what is wrong with your life and take steps to change. Of course, many people think that they do not need to change or do not need someone to help them look at themselves from the other perspectives.

Mentally, of course, people can work on their attitude. This is very difficult since there is rampant fear and often anger, the anger that accompanies any strong condition, or disease: anger at God, anger at others, anger at self. So, controlling the mind is of utmost importance. And again, it is difficult while one is in the throes of this condition. This condition is in charge. So, again, seek help. *Let others help you.*

Spiritually, when one has AIDS, it is a time for introspection, a time to examine one's life and the decisions that one has run life with, and a time to change those decisions about life, if possible. It is a time to just think quietly inside oneself. As with all diseases, one gets plenty of quiet time by oneself. But this may not necessarily be good thinking time, because the disease is in charge.

Often, it is at this time when the *will* gets kicked into action, which is the most important factor in fighting the disease. It is necessary for the person who has manifestations of the disease to find enough will to care for themselves to fight the enemy, the virus. One simply must fight for oneself and learn about power and strength in a wise way. One can harness one's will, spiritually, as an energy force within oneself. Just search for it in introspection and find it.

3

Antidotes To Fear

Own Your Own Fears To Release Them

Master Adalfo

You have noticed that many people have been exhibiting anger about this disease. Some want to keep their children out of school. Their anger is a *cover-up* for fear. People are afraid. One way to deal with that fear is first to *own* the feeling they have that they are afraid they will get AIDS. That's really what is involved. People don't say it, they don't admit that fear. If you don't admit being fearful, how can you deal with it? If you say, "I am afraid for my child, or other children," that is not owning the fact that you are afraid for yourself. Really, the fear is about you.

First of all, people need to face the fear that they are afraid of acquiring the disease themselves because at the moment it means death. They are afraid of dying. So, if people begin to own that feeling, it is easier to pass from judgment about it into a way of dealing with it. If you pretend it is something else, then you cannot face it or deal with it because it isn't real, it's something else. So, people must first experience and acknowledge (which is what I really mean by owning) that this is a gut feeling. What they are afraid of is dying, and they are particularly afraid of dying of the disease that has the stigma this one has.

Once they acknowledge this, they can face other areas in their life in which they have been afraid. They can begin to look at why they are afraid of dying. What is dying to them? What has dying meant in their lives? What has it meant to them when a parent died, when a pet died, when a beautiful bouquet of flowers has died? What does that mean to them? Does that mean God is depriving them again, and is this another instance of lack? Does it mean that they are sad because they do not have this person or this bouquet of flowers in their life? Does it mean they are unable to see the abundance for the flowers or for that person who passes on to a happier, fuller, richer, plane of existence?

People must begin to see the beauty, the abundance there is in life, but they will have to face their fear of death first. They will have to do this and they will have to say, "I am afraid of dying." People are so afraid they won't even say they are fearful of death. You find some people who do not make a will because they think they don't *need* it. Instead of saying, "I'm afraid of dying, I don't want to make a will. That would mean I will die," they make up other excuses. People have to begin to be honest, starting with self.

Do not judge yourself harshly for having a fear of death, and do not be judging others who have the disease or the fear. Once you own a feeling that you have, how can you judge anyone else for having the same feeling? You will not rush to judge others if you know you have the same feeling, the same situation. Judgment comes when you believe you are exempt from such feelings. And self-judgment is the same thing. If you believe you ought to be exempt from such feelings, then you will judge yourself harshly for having it instead of saying, "Ah, I have it, now what?" Feelings just are. They are not logical. They cannot be judged.

Often they don't make any sense, that is true. And sometimes people say, "I shouldn't have it because it doesn't make any sense." That isn't true, they have it. They choose to *not act* on it because it doesn't make sense. That's a different thing. That's owning the feeling first and then saying, "OK, that's how I feel, but I don't have to act on that feeling." The mark of a mature adult is that they have the feeling, but don't act on it, they chose to do something differently.

There are many ways to deal with a deep feeling. One way is to

131

talk to someone. Another way is to write it down and create a comfortable little ceremony. You may wish to write it down and bury it in the ground as a giveaway, giving away your fear. You may write it down and watch it burn. Someone we know uses the game of soap bubbles. He encases what he no longer wishes to have in a bubble and blows it away. So each person must find their own ceremony. What you are doing is giving your fear away to the Universe which can transform it to become just energy again. Instead of being negative energy, it just becomes energy which can then be positively used.

Enid

Fear has so many different levels to it. But the unreasoning fear is when that fear hits the rock bottom part of you, and no matter how hard you try, you can't get rid of it. You can even talk to yourself and say, "No, I shouldn't be feeling this much afraid, and I'm ashamed of myself for feeling this way." Well, that's the *deep unreasoning fear* and it's part of the physical universe. It is a very, very strong portion of what we call "fear." And it turns on when there are life-threatening situations. The interesting part is that many of the people who suffer from this unreasoning fear are not anywhere near those with AIDS. They don't know anyone who has AIDS. Perhaps they're not even in a part of the country where it's showing up, and yet they feel this terrible fear inside themselves.

For every emotion that we feel, the *deeper* we're willing to feel that emotion, the more we're going to get out of the experience. That's small comfort for someone who can't seem to still that terrible, fearful anxiety in the pit of the stomach or around the solar plexus. Deep breathing is one of the best ways to help that because when one is caught in the grips of fear, oxygen is denied to the head and the fear begins to grow and grow as more and more oxygen is denied. So deep breathing, in through the nose and out through the mouth, is very good to help dispel the worst part of it.

We are sympathetic here about what you go through in your emotional experiences, but this too, my darlings, is *just another emotional experience*. There is another and very interesting part to it,

132

however. It is turned on by certain symbols. And it's almost as though they're electrically connected. There's a network of these feelings that just sweep the country or just sweep the world, and one of those symbols has to do with radiation. If you'll notice, in the very last stages of the experience of AIDS, it's very similar to what those who suffer from radiation poisoning experience; the changing of the body cell and the growing of it in an almost cancerous kind of way. And that symbol of bombing, that symbol of life threat for all of life, is what has triggered this unreasoning fear. And you know, the bottom line to that (in the physical universe) is being afraid of dying.

Understand that nobody dies. But we do have to have some way of getting rid of our bodies when the time comes, you see? The fear of death is so excruciating, especially the fear of terrible, slow death–awful feelings of that–it's that unreasoning fear that you can't explain to yourself even. And it grips you and you can't let it go.

Now deep breathing will help a lot, but the emotion is there to be experienced. *It's there to be experienced.* And for those of you who have that fear and do experience that fear, the first thing I would ask you to do is to stop judging yourself for it. Stop judging yourself for the way you're feeling, and allow that feeling to take its full course. You understand that any emotion is going to magnify when you're trying to turn it off. So instead of trying to get away from that fear, allow yourself to feel it right in your heart and solar plexus. Say, "All right, I want to feel this fear as hard as I possibly can. I want to feel it. I want to experience and I don't want to run away from it because it's a gift, it's a message from the physical Universe. It's a message from my Higher Self. It's a deep, deep strong feeling which brings the greatest of rewards."

So, allow yourself to feel it as strongly as you possibly can, taking away all the resistance. Please understand, dear heart, it's the resistance that's making it harder for you. So don't hold it back. Allow yourself to feel it. "I want to feel more fear now, come on, come on, feel it now." Put your hand across your heart and solar plexus, saying, "Come on fear, grip me harder, I want to feel you." And you'll find it easing. You'll find it easing away, easing away. And you can use the energy in the same way as we tell those with AIDS to use the energy–

to propel themselves into a new state of consciousness. You see, the person with that terrible fear gripping them, is experiencing AIDS in a spiritual way, in an emotional way.

So there's a lot of mileage that's coming out of this disease, believe you me, a lot of things are happening. And when it's all over with, we can review it. We can look back and we can see all of the richness that occurred as a result of this incredible virus. And we can see parts of it being a gift for us. We can see how that fear drove us into a higher point, into a bigger place, a place where we can see things in a new way and experience life in a greater way. We've talked about experiencing all these deep things and the great reward. Well, there's a reward here, a certain confidence that builds up in you, a certain feeling of confidence when you have paid your dues. So be comforted, my darlings, all is not lost. Even in your fear, you are winning the game.

See Your Perfection

Kyros

Within the mass consciousness of the Earth, some illnesses have been designated as being incurable. This is only your relative truth based on your lack of understanding of the Universal laws and principles and your lack of spiritual awareness. As you ascend into understanding and grow in awareness, you will then realize that All is Perfection.

When Jesus performed what you consider to be His miraculous acts of healing, He was seeing perfection of form, as opposed to disease-ridden bodies or crippled and deformed limbs. When He told a man to take up his bed and walk, He saw a perfect form, not a crippled one. He commanded with authority. He did not beg, pamper or plead and He did not take the suffering onto Himself. He worked with the spiritual, mental and emotional levels of the patient and when these were touched, the physical responded. The great element in His healing work was that of complete and total love. No one can heal or be an instrument of complete healing unless these two things

134

are present: *seeing the one to be healed as perfect, and loving that person totally and completely.*

If you happen to be in need of healing, there are some things you can do to assist in your own healing. Physicians, holistic doctors, psychic healers and so forth are but instruments to help you trigger your *own healing energies* into action. The Christ would trigger the healing energies in others by the touch of His hand or a word, but always He saw perfection of form. He was a channel of total love.

You can assist in your own healing by seeing yourself as perfect and by loving yourself totally and completely. This assists the healing instrument (whatever or however it may happen to you) to help you. If you are filled with negativity or doubt, you can block your own healing energies. It is also critical that you examine your own emotional and mental levels. To be healed and to remain healed, one must make changes in his life experience. One cannot remain healed if one continues to hold negative thoughts and attitudes. If the emotional and mental levels are not dealt with, the healing is not complete. When the spiritual, mental, and emotional levels are brought into calmness, balance, and joy, then the physical will respond. It *has to respond* because it is not what you, in essence, are. You are perfect Spirit, not an imperfect form.

It is only your ego which keeps trying to convince you how imperfect and fragile you and others are. It keeps you centered on the imperfection of yourself and others. In doing so, it keeps you imprisoned by the illusions of sickness, despair, death, and chaos. All entities can be channels for healing, but they must first raise their levels of awareness in order to see perfection in All and they must love. Start first with yourself.

As the Master Christ said, "Physician, heal thyself!" So also do I say this to you, *"See the perfection of your own creation and love your own creation."* Remember that you have been created by and out of the Lord Most High and if you do not love yourself, you are denying love to your Creator. Once you love yourself and see your own perfection, you can no longer see others as imperfect and you will love all men and all creation. You are then completely healed and can become a true channel of healing for others.

135

Find Calmness Within

Ting-Lao

The fear is great and when there is fear, oftentimes the Spirit body, the Spirit self, cannot get into the physical body to influence the personality and to calm the fear. It is a cycle. So, just sitting in calmness is good. This is one thing that is easier to do when one is sick. But, do not sit in fear. Use this time constructively. I know this is hard, but one must pull up this fighting discipline and do these different kinds of things. Just to be sitting with oneself, just to be feeling oneself, just to be intending to know oneself, doesn't require so much effort. It doesn't require that you do things with your mind or listen to meditation tapes, but just that you be *with* yourself.

Oftentimes, people are so busy, busy doing so many things in the world that they do not invest time and energy in just being with themselves. By doing so, however, they will discover many things about themselves that will be very healing and very enjoyable and they will have a new relationship with themselves that will give them strength to put aside this fear. There is no need to fight the fear; rather, people need to put it aside. Just say, "Oh, that is fear. I feel it. I felt it." Then breathe deeply and put it aside. There is no big battle or fight or lesson here, except to step aside from it, to let it be.

4

The Immune System

Create Your Own Truths

Zoosh

AIDS is merely an outgrowth of many breakdowns in the immunological system as a means for all of you to understand that you have the power to *create your own immunology* in your thoughts, beliefs, and emotions. For those of you who have decided to participate in the mutating forms of the AIDS symptomatology, understand that this is a challenge of your own ability to move beyond what others tell you is the truth. Your body contains everything within it that is needed to move beyond any form of disease. Yes, your body can do this.

If you believe you have one, you have an immunological system. If you believe that it is a hot day, you can step outside where everybody is wearing snow boots. You can observe that there is funny white stuff coming down, and the people are throwing it around and having a good time and are wearing mufflers and heavy clothes. You can be wearing shorts, and still be warm in the cold. Conversely, you can be cool and comfortable in hot.

It is the ability *not* to deny the truth of others, but instead to create your *own truth* within your own comfort zone, bringing the spiritual inspiration into the material plane—the *now* into the linear life. Linear refers to a time continuum. Now is absolute time, wherein right now, everything is happening and all knowledge and power are

137

available to you—right now.

It is for you to know, if you are going to move beyond this disease that while the immunological system within your physical self is being attacked on many fronts, you can create physical evidence to reflect why it is being attacked. You really can alter your symptomatology. I would suggest, in the face of physical evidence to the contrary, that you believe that you are healthy; just as the person might believe that, while walking around in the snow drifts, they are warm and exhibit signs of warmth (and you have seen evidence that this can exist). *Change your mind, change your life.*

Allow yourself to be in that moment. It can be done, but you will have to fly in the face of the physical evidence that is within yourself for the time. You may not receive much respect and support from those around you for your way of treating your disease. I'm not saying to deny yourself medical care in its conventional forms. I am saying to *add* to that your change of attitude and your absolute belief in your own body's ability to reject all forms of discomfort. See yourself being attracted to health and comfort. And in time, move beyond the idea of rejecting disease and *move toward the idea of accepting* health.

Getting In Touch With Your Own Heart

Dong How Li

What is going to increase the production of cells that are willing to fight, able to fight, know what to fight? I ask you. Do you have any ideas? Getting back in touch with the heart is a good place to start, since it circulates the blood in your body and the antibodies that fight for you. The thymus gland, which rules the immune system, is associated with and placed behind the heart. If you nourish your hearts by finding ways of filling them with such things as *what you do* and *who you are with,* these things will increase and fill you. They will give you the will to live, the desire to live, and you will find that you have what is *needed* to fight off what is inappropriate for you. But when your heart is weak and you are not feeding it that which makes it full and whole, then you are not tending to it. Soon you will find that

138

you do not have much will to live, and because of this, it will be hard for you to fight off that which could kill you.

Love Yourself And Others

Zoosh

For those of you who have experienced this disease in its many forms, begin now, on an emotional level, to experience only love for yourself and your world. When you catch yourself being depressed, know that even though you may have very good reasons to be depressed, it will only serve to make things more uncomfortable for you. Now, even though it may require you to look at your world completely differently, be cheerful! Know in yourself that your sense of good feeling about yourself and your cheeriness will help you to change disease.

Understand that positivity and lovingness is common throughout your Universe, but not yet common on this planet. So, realize that the cure to this disease, as well as to all diseases, is to remain totally loving of yourself, totally accepting and allowing of yourself and others. Remain cheerful and happy on an emotional level, and don't deny those things which have upset you. Be experiencing and acting out physically, as well as emotionally, true love and happiness for yourself. This is the cure. It is also, perhaps, a better demonstration than discomfort. Pat yourselves on the back and say, *"I've been involved in a great movement to show the world that love is all right."* And begin now to love yourself and to know that you have *done well.*

Taulmus

For those individuals who have contracted AIDS and who are of homosexual persuasion, it is most important that you learn not to judge yourselves. The choice that you have made to love another of your own gender is not wrong or bad as the worldly view would have it. Living with public judgment of your *chosen* life-style and being unsure yourselves of the rightness of your choice has set up a

139

defensive and fearful pattern in your thinking, which has left you wide open for this new disease that now flourishes on your land. Also, the babble of the news media and the fervor of the press has done more of a disservice than it has assisted anyone. Fear is catching.

To give up judgment of yourself necessitates that you forgive *imagined* wrongs and evil deeds. I say imagined because, from where I sit, there is not the duality of right and wrong, good or bad, but merely the expressing of All That Is. Man created the should's and the should not's, the laws, and then called these laws pronouncements of a God on high who rules your world with a stern and unbending force. So, give up judgment of yourselves and your fellow beings and know that the highest service that you can do to your soul is *to love* the grand person that you are.

There seems to be much confusion in your world as to what it truly means, this love of one's self. Love of self means that *your* comfort and *your* peace of mind must always come *first* with you. When you have achieved a balance within your own energy field, when you have nourished yourself, *only* then can you have an abundance of love to share with another.

Love of self does not mean the cultivation of the false vanity that presently appears to be at an all-time high on your plane. This is when the clothes that one adorns themselves, the hair arrangement, the car that is driven and the home that is lived in, become a total preoccupation. Love of self does not mean that you allow others to manipulate you to do their bidding. Self-sacrifice has wrongly been thought of as a spiritual attribute when, in truth, it is a degrading experience for all concerned. Love of self, very simply put, is your knowledge and awareness of who you are as a multi-dimensional, unlimited being, and the realization of your importance in the larger scheme of things. *How could you not love such a being?* Be aware that as you each learn love of self, it is then that you give all others who you come in contact with, the encouragement and permission to love themselves. That is a high purpose, to be sure.

So, give up judgment and learn to love. This is for *all* beings. Those who have loved ones stricken with AIDS need especially to work on these things. For often it is the embarrassment of a parent or sibling who has judged that particular member of their family who has chosen to live the unconventional life of a homosexual which is the core of the problem.

Enid

There is a reminder here that there is great value in loving one another, rather than being animals with one another, if you understand the difference. That is not a judgment, but an observation. You can deal with the sexual part of you, shoving it away from you and doing only the animal part of it and enjoying only that, or you can go deeper into your experience and enjoy a deeper experience with it. This is not to say that those who have AIDS have not done this, but definitely those who are afraid that they may get AIDS are beginning to look at their sexuality differently. They're beginning to see that it's an extension of love and expression rather than an animal activity. So, there is a greater consciousness arising there.

The raising of consciousness does not mean that homosexuals are deciding not to be homosexual because most beings are born with that proclivity. Some change afterwards, but for the most part, beings are born with that intent. So, they must live that out until they decide otherwise or not. It is never the question that we must bring them to an understanding that they should become like "the rest of us" or to be heterosexual, but rather to point out that greater waves of loving exist that do not involve the physical, animal-type experience. There is a greater consciousness of the act of loving being more important than the animal activity. Very definitely.

You know that the reason for AIDS isn't to teach homosexuals a lesson. It's just that it took hold in that community much more easily because there was a greater changing of partners. This doesn't occur among most heterosexuals because they tend to stay with one person longer.

Creating A Comfort Zone

Zoosh

You will find, now, that if you reject your fellow beings who are exhibiting signs of this AIDS disease, that you will only be rejecting your own ability to maintain your health and comfort, for the AIDS situation is about comfort and discomfort. You will be rejecting your own ability to maintain comfort regardless of the situation. And everyone *does* have the ability to maintain comfort and to create a comfort zone, regardless of the situation. This is how some people can walk on hot coals. They create a sense of comfort and a belief in their ability to do anything to prove to themselves, as well as to the world, that they can go beyond the laws of physical evidence.

So, I'm not suggesting that you walk over hot coals or walk through fire. I am saying that in order to believe in your abilities, in order to enhance your own feminine energy (for both men and women) you will need to allow your inspiration, which will come from your soul self, to be expanded upon by your imagination, which will come from your mind self. You will need to make the leap across the so-called "rainbow bridge" (where there is no obvious physical substance) to know that you will be safe.

So, know that you are safe in all circumstances. You can *generate your own safety* by feeling secure in who you are and by knowing that this disease is not something you will incorporate in your life. It is that simple.

5

Finding Your Heart

Caring

Dong How Li

All healing is self-healing, whether you do that with crystals or with others who are assisting you in the process as priest, as healer, as therapist, as friend. What you are attempting to do in the process of healing is to bring all the parts of you back into harmony again, to reinstitute communication you have allowed to disconnect through the processes of fear, of self-loathing, of disappointment, or of loss.

Operating in the field where inside is outside and outside is inside, your healer then becomes the projected part of you, the Higher Self projected, enabling you to put your pieces back together. This is the work of priesthood, and since priesthood is no longer in good favor, you have many other names for it nowadays—acupuncture is one of these. As you reconnect these parts of yourself within your being, you will notice they are also reconnected in your life. You will notice relationships change. You will read the signs of life around you and their messages to you more clearly.

Now, in the western tradition of Judeo-Christianity, the focus has been primarily outer. Sometimes this works. But if you will notice, more and more it is failing. People are turning to more traditional ways of healing, more natural ways of healing which require they go inside. And in case you haven't already noticed, the planet, and what is going on within it, around it and on it, is now forcing everyone, more and more, to go inside.

Many, many more people will be forced, by disease (if they don't accept the messages sooner), or circumstances, or relationships, to go deeper within, and to go deeper faster. It is not going to be so difficult as you all learn to move in that direction, especially as you all center in your hearts. My favorite image about the heart is that, as you learn to center there, it is easier to move because it is always with you. Your center is always with you wherever you go. And no matter how topsy-turvy the world gets, or how much the ground shakes, you spin like a top from this center.

So, much of how I discuss healing has to do with *finding one's heart,* has to do with learning what moves you, what inspires you, what recharges you, what gives you energy, as opposed to depleting you, exhausting you, raising fear within you. This plague you are calling AIDS is a *massive broken heart.* It is no mistake, in almost all of your so-called "civilized" countries, heart disease is on incredible increase. People don't know what their hearts are, where they are, figuratively or literally. Believe me, one does not find one's heart by getting a plastic one. So, in some ways, that is going off on the wrong track.

One must begin to find within oneself what moves one, what inspires one. With the energy of that, one has enough to move the thymus gland to reactivate and regenerate the immune system to increase circulation inside and outside and improve health.

You will hear other teachers from other traditions speak in other ways, but if you look underneath, they will also be speaking about the heart, the going inward. Has it not also been said in your tradition of Christianity, that the second coming will be in your hearts? *This is that time,* my friends. It is already upon you. And it is intensifying.

So, how *does* one find one's heart, how does one use medicine, how does one use the arts, how does one use stones, plants, and other people to find one's heart, to heal oneself? One must first open up to being human and to feeling because only through one's feelings (second chakra) and heart (fourth chakra) do you have the gateway open to the third eye (sixth chakra) which is insight. And only with

144

feeling will you know where your heart is leading. This is a major turnaround for this culture which would prefer to be led with its mind. But, of course, it is obvious where that has led. The destruction is rampant and everywhere.

Many people now are finding they *have* to deal with their emotional body, all of these feelings, and that is exactly what's going to be intensifying. You will notice you will get angrier more often. You also are going to notice that many people are angry more often. This is going to be projected outward because they think it is easier to deal with it outside of themselves than inside themselves. But that only perpetuates the problem. Better they should go inside and deal with it and not have to project their anger toward others.

There is going to be a lot of this kind of polarization. It is already starting. And you must watch for it within yourselves. You must watch your own flip-flops in mood, in opinion, in willingness to take responsibility. It's going to be *very challenging*. But, you have all *chosen* to be here at this time, not only for the lessons, but for the talent and the leadership you have to offer. As you know, the planet is wounded and in need of healing, and as you help yourselves, you help her and all beings upon her.

To encourage this healing process within yourselves and among others and on the planet, one goes inward, one works with one's heart. One uses whatever tools are available. However, at this time it is tricky because people get hung up on the tools. Remember that your point is to find your heart. So yes, you may use red stones. Yes, you may use beautiful string music that opens up your heart. You may do improvisational movements. You may find other people such as psychotherapists to work with you. There are many ways, all valid. And before you are through, you may use them all, depending on where you are at any one point and time.

What you are trying to do is to *open your hearts primarily to yourselves*. You know, Christianity is marvelous. It is so outer directed, when everything Christ was doing was *inner directed*. So, now you are trying to open up despite the fear, and allow your heart to feel and to breathe and to receive and to give.

Healing, my friends, is the free movement of this whole part (the

145

heart) of your being. You will notice, if you look at many people in the streets and around you in different places, you will find many with hunched shoulders, hiding their hearts and protecting them, running from them, even from themselves which not only keeps other people out, but keeps themselves out. It is most curious. Truly the heart is your treasure. It is the seat of all of your healing powers. It is the transformer. It takes everything from below, cleanses, and offers it up. Everything from above is given down, everything from all directions moves from the heart.

As you work with finding your hearts, finding what is there, finding where you want to go, finding what the blocks are that are keeping you from where you want to go, you will breathe more space, more air and allowance, you will find it easier to share.

Master Adalfo

Healing is loving and loving is healing. So, when we do anything which is an act of caring or an act of love, that is healing. When someone loves us, we are healed by that love. So any modality, *anything* that produces that loving or caring or nurtured feeling is healing. Some doctors are real healers because they have that special caring, loving energy; some are not, because they do not. That is what healing is. It is not just skill, although skill helps. It is the loving and the caring that heals.

Believing

Soli

Love is unconditional acceptance, total and unconditional. It is the way of the new society. It is the way of the Aquarian Age—*no judgments*. The more you learn not to judge, the more you will find yourself not being judged by others, because whatever you believe about yourself is what everybody around you will see. It doesn't matter what the physical body looks like. If you believe it is ugly, it will be ugly to others. If you believe it is beautiful, if you constantly

146

see the beauty that you are and manifest that, this is what others will see in you. *Beliefs*, my friends, especially self-beliefs, *create your realities.*

Disease is not necessary if you follow your inner guidance, if you find and make contact with your Higher Self. Do not judge those who find themselves with a disease. It is a natural state of being for the human upon the Earth plane. Once you have totally transcended the subconscious mind, then you have no need to be upon the Earth plane any longer. You then have finished your lives here, for you have learned all there is to learn about the power of creation through thought.

Everything that is, is a thought in the mind of God. Everything that you are is a thought in that *part of God that you are.* So do not judge others; have compassion, my friends, not pity. For pity says, "I see what you are and I think you should be something different and I feel sorry for you. It is a great pity that you are not something else." That is judgment, my friends. How can you look at another's life and judge it and say they should not be doing what they are doing?

Compassion, on the other hand, says, "You are human. I am human, too. Therefore I know what you are experiencing. I know what you are going through. I know what you are creating for yourself and why, and I accept your right to do that. I will help you in any way that I can, but I will not interfere or judge you for what you are *right now.*"

You can cure any illness if you understand the communication behind it and take action upon that communication and turn it around. Those who have AIDS can turn it around if they work hard and long enough, and truly learn to love self and learn to take responsibility for self. For many, however, it is a socially acceptable form of suicide. And that is all right, too. For everyone ultimately leaves the Earth plane some way or another. This is just one of the many ways.

There will always be viruses and germs and other kinds of bugs available to help you. If you have an infection, and understand the communication behind it, you bless the little bugs that have given you that help, that communication. Thank them, send them your love and tell them you don't need them any longer. They will go, almost

147

instantly, if you have understood the communication and taken action.

If you have apparently cured that illness by mechanical means, and you have *not understood* the communication, it will return sooner or later. But once you have understood the communication, taken action, made the necessary changes in your life and taken the responsibility for your own life, the bugs will disappear. They will go somewhere else, for they are living Spirits, too, as is every single thing upon this Earth plane.

6

Using Your Emotions

Zoosh

Speaking primarily to those who are exhibiting symptomology or who believe they may have AIDS, use your power to create. Use your emotions, right now! *Use your emotions.* The emotions have always been ascribed to the feminine. So specifically speaking to the masculine beings right now, it is time to be emotional. When you hear you have the disease, cry, scream, yell, do all of that. That will be the beginning of your healing.

Now, I'm not saying you have to rush around and break dishes and go crazy. What I am saying is that you need to allow your emotional self to express itself with as much honor as you have given to your mental self. Your mental self right now calculates and controls and does not allow your physical self to be its natural, joyous counterpart.

So I would suggest that for a time, you allow yourself to be *totally emotional.* If something strikes you funny, do not go "heeheehee," go "HAHAHAHA." Allow yourself to be highly charged emotionally. This will help you to be inspired. Spirit energy and emotionality, which links inspiration to the physical self, are the two aspects of yourselves that you need to incorporate more now.

So the theme is *action* on the emotional front. I would suggest that if you are angry, that you do not control yourself. The time for control is over. I'm not suggesting that you go out and punch somebody in the

149

nose. I am suggesting that you go into your bedroom and you have one heck of a temper tantrum. Get mad at the world, punch your pillow, throw it against the wall, or if you can go out on the land, even better. You just yell and scream and feel sorry for yourself, do whatever it takes.

If you are mobile, go out on the land some place and stand on the ground. Get yourself a heavy stick, ask the ground's permission (make sure you're not poking any rabbit holes) and have yourself a temper tantrum by standing on the land. The land's energy will come through you in ways that you will not understand until you are done. When you are done you will know you are done because you will begin to laugh.

Understand the purpose of having a tantrum is not to just get back at the world and feel sorry for yourself (which is all right), but to allow your emotional energies, which are the *link* between the Spirit and the physical, to run *through* you. And you will know that you have completed this process when you feel the energy moving from the Earth through your feet and simultaneously up and down the body. You will know the feeling. You will be rejoicing within you. It will be your Mother the planet, rejoicing within you for allowing yourself to receive the truth of the Mother (Spirit-Mother-Earth) energies. Normally, in your controlling aspects, you will not allow that energy to flow easily. So, once you purge yourself of your immediate anger and rage, allow yourself to laugh about it. Don't force it. If the laughter comes naturally, allow it to be. And in that sense you will find that the purpose of the anger exercise is to allow yourself to be that emotional being in the positive sense. When you hear something funny after that (and it won't take much to get you to laugh), you will laugh more outwardly without trying to control it.

The time for control has come to an end. And the time of spontaneity, happiness, and joy is here, but you must honor your emotions, you need to do that. Your emotions may test you. They might create conditions for you, such as a belief in a disease, by giving you the apparent symptoms of any disease. It could be a cold. It doesn't have to be anything so dramatic as AIDS.

You can check around inside your physical self. Are there any places of tightness there? Is there any restriction, any stress, anything you're holding back? If so, that would be the time to go out to the land and have that anger exercise again. Use that stick and beat the ground. Yell and scream. Say anything you want. Make sure you're by yourself. Yell and scream and curse everybody out. Don't try and be logical. Don't think, "Well, there's no reason to be mad at them, they've never done anything to me." Just let it out. Understand that logic is control.

Now I'm not saying that logic is the enemy. I'm not saying that the mind is the enemy. I am merely saying that your mind has been overly stimulated and has been too much a part of your life. So, right now, understand that we are talking about the pathway from discomfort to comfort, which is the goal of any being on this planet.

Use your physical self. When you feel comfort inside your physical self, you will know that you have attained a natural state of being. When you feel tightness anywhere, then you will know that you need to do something physical. You need to honor the physical plane and do something physical. Get angry, go out and run, do something stimulating and see if that tightness goes away. If it doesn't go away, then you will need to have the anger exercise again (or something like it), in order to honor your need to purge yourself of your negative emotions. They are not logical so they will not come out in a logical way. Do not force them to be logical. If your emotions were logical you would not be able to communicate with them in these new ways. You would be able to control them as you have done with your mind.

151

7

Awaken Your Energies

Ting-Lao

We must awaken the energies of the body. Most people today, in all walks of life, are too complacent with their lives and have become stagnant. You people must wake up and bring yourself to full consciousness. Get more sleep so you can wake up more refreshed and live life with more vigor, more energy. This is the key to raising your vibrations, which will enable you to lift yourself out of illness. Illness is not necessary.

Getting together with people is also important. People live in relationship to other people; that is part of being in a body. So, active human relationships are important. Don't isolate yourselves so much. Isolation is boring. Many people watch too much television, living in a fantasy world there, instead of actively getting together with other people.

Do more exercises, get your prana (life-force energy) flowing. Too many people are tired. We encourage everyone to become active to prevent the spread of AIDS, to prevent the spread of illness, by living life more vigorously and with full participation.

Remember also, the energy field around the Earth is vitally important in any disease, but particularly in this disease of AIDS because this is the only way to get enough power to encapsulate and overcome the actual physical entities of the virus in the body. It must be done with much, much power from this earth energy, channeling this energy up through one's body to keep oneself strong, to prevent it from succumbing to the virus, and to heal it. This is the way to heal it on a physical level. You can kill the virus in the body with such a vibration of energy from the Earth that the molecules of the virus cannot exist, cannot migrate, and must fall apart, must disintegrate. This is the physical way.

The emotional way to heal the person is by raising the consciousness, the introspection, and bonding with oneself. When these changes are made, then the disease entityness cannot form again, cannot re-form, and it stays disintegrated. Do not think it is a disease that we cannot conquer.

By not keeping oneself full of light and life, one allows the entityness of the disease to have a place to grow and live. If you do not clean in the corners, the mold and fungus can grow because there is no light or cleanliness. So too, one must have light and awareness and cleanliness in the body and in the consciousness so that these diseases do not get in. This is one of the reasons why some people succumb to the virus in their bodies and other people may go for years without succumbing—they have more life force in their bodies.

So, what we need to do is just not give the virus a place to live. We must say, "I understand that you have a prime directive, you are an entityness, you do need to live. So go away. Go live on some other planet, go live in some other realm or energy dimension. Go where your disease lives. It may not live in this body." There is no reason to accept the virus. This is not a necessary way of learning lessons. People fall into disease through laziness, unconsciousness and unawareness because they are not progressing on their own. They need to get this "kick in the rear." However, I want the people to know that it is not a *necessary* way of learning or progressing in the human culture.

Dong How Li

Remember, emotion is energy. You can go with that flow and allow it to expand itself. And, indeed, in that way you can use it to get where you want to be. Crying is very important. Laughing is very

153

important. Deep breathing is very important. Movement is very important to keep your energy moving. People are so concerned about aging. Aging is an attempt to stop the flow. Aging is the accumulation of innumerable stops of the flow. What you want to do is to keep moving, keep the energy inside you moving.

Health, like love, like truth, is about owning more and more of you, not disowning, not separating, not disconnecting. I like to think, in my tradition, that all sin is an act of separation, at any level, from the rest of your life—your heart from your feet. Thus, any act of separation is a lie.

Health does not only involve the body but it involves the emotions, the mind and the Spirit as well. So, therefore, every disease has all of these components. All these aspects of your being are involved in everything that manifests in you, even if it only manifests in the physical, even if it only manifests in the emotional. So, then, to the degree that you deal with all these aspects, you can accelerate the healing of a specific problem.

I encourage you, in your meditations, to please sit and just list the activities you *enjoy* doing, even those that you don't have the time for, that you don't have the money for, that you can't do from where you are now, even those. All of them must be affirming to your health. (I am not affirming cocaine habits; you know, these days, one must qualify.) Some people believe because they enjoy something, it is all right. But, we want what affirms *all* of you: body, emotions, mind, and Spirit. Collect those, list those, and then begin to see what you can give yourself, a little at a time, a little more, and a little more, and a little more.

8

Communicating With
Your
Higher Self

Meditation And Visualization

Soli

When disease comes along, contact your Higher Self through meditation. Ask the Higher Self, "What is it that you wish me to do? What is the communication behind this? What is it that I am not facing? What is it that I am not living up to?"

Various parts of the body have various and different logical aspects. Some of the common phraseology pertaining to this has a lot of common sense. For example, we refer to the heart as the "center of love." We say a person is "sticking his nose into somebody's business." If you have an illness or disease of the lower extremities, you are obviously being "slowed down" because you will not slow yourself down any other way. If you have difficulty standing up straight, you are "not facing the world." From these various aspects, you will find what the true communication is. Once you have understood the communication, then you take action to make the necessary changes. Sometimes, people actually prefer having the disease to making the changes. They prefer to leave the Earth plane rather than make the changes they must make in order to continue here. And it is always free will and choice. Understand the communication and take action.

Ultimately, meditation centers the subconscious mind and allows the energy of the Higher Self to come through. If you have totally centered that subconscious mind, you will have a feeling of energy, of light, and great vibration awakens around you. That is the energy of the Higher Self coming through. Meditation is simply centering the subconscious mind, withdrawing your consciousness from the five senses and allowing it to be in contact with your spiritual self, the Higher Self.

Visualization is the most common and the most popular means of centering, for visualizing some object keeps the subconscious mind busy. Guided meditations and creative visualizations are also valuable. It is a form of hypnosis, self-hypnosis. Of course, all hypnosis is self-hypnosis, for you have to *do it yourself.* You have to follow the instructions. And so it is this centering of the subconscious, getting it out of the way, that allows the energy of the Higher Self to come through.

Dr. Peebles

Visualize, in your daily meditation, a white light flowing through your entire system from your feet to your head. Visualize this light flowing up the tributaries into your blood stream, so that your blood stream itself is carrying particles of light, so that any darkness it finds is gathered up and released into that light. Then visualize the light flushing everything that is not in harmony, not in balance and not of total right action out of your body. It will help keep your physical strength in harmony. It will help you with keeping a balanced weight. It will keep you young and youthful-looking. It will keep you in harmony with your personality, with your soul, and with the masters. Understand that the light and energy flows into all of you, automatically. However, through improper physical diet, through improper mental diet, through the lack of daily meditation and affirmation, most of that light and energy is dissipated, which, in turn, creates your symptoms.

If you have a particular disease, let's say cancer, then visualize those cells surrounded in the white light and picture a snapping little clam entering that light and gobbling up all the cells. When the clam is full, release it from your body. You can visualize a ray gun

156

destroying all those cells in the light. Whatever works for you, use it to work within your body. Cleanse that negativity. If, however, you have done everything possible, then you must understand that this disease is karmic for you, and it is not for you to heal on a physical level.

Visualization is a mental process. When you visualize your body to be perfect, and you heal yourself, do not take this to the physical level and start bragging, or saying that you are a perfect being or any of that. This would attract the illnesses back to you. When you start expressing this verbally, you are demonstrating the personality of this life and you are taking away from your power. You must *live it and demonstrate it through the example of your life.*

Sleep Programming

Dr. Peebles

When you enter the period of sleep, if you have released your day and dealt with your experiences, you blend them with all facets of yourself (physically, mentally, emotionally, and spiritually) so that your Higher Self is the controlling factor, rather than your conscious self. It is equal to being on the Spirit side, where you put things into their balances and proper perspectives. By doing this and practicing toward it, your Higher Self becomes clear and strong and will bring about the healing of your sets of circumstances. In some cases, it will be done in one hour of sleep; in others, after a series of nights.

Also remember that if you are in a situation that you know is not one you must hold onto, and you have not found the healing technique in your sleep, if you have not found energy sources on your conscious levels, then project astrally to the realm of the psychic healer, the psychic surgeons. You will have psychic surgery and you will be healed. Obviously, you must have tremendous faith in yourself. You must trust that your body and your mind are within your control as a total being and that there is nothing that will obsess or possess you.

So, if you approach sleep as a time for growth and balance and prepare yourself for it with that knowledge and belief, then, indeed,

157

you will experience growth, and healing will automatically take place. I think it is sometimes far better than going to the healers themselves.

Ting-Lao

In ancient Egypt, and other cultures, dream work consisted of doing what you now call "programming dreams" or lucid dreaming. This is where you go into the dream world knowing that it is a real place. Just as you can step into your sixth chakra in meditation practice as a real place, you can step into the dream world, which is the astral plane. At night you live there just as you live in the physical world when you are awake. Many people come to the point where they feel they are living 24 hours a day. They make the physical body rest at night and then they come into the physical body (from the astral) in the morning. It is a great opportunity to help smooth out life in a physical body, to use that time to do work, just as you would do work on this world during the daylight hours.

To begin the practice of working with your dreams, start with the positioning of the head. This will have certain effects on the dreams. You may want to experiment with facing the head in the different directions of north, east, south, or west.

Then channel energy up through the feet before you go to sleep. First pull the toes back toward your head and flex the feet, pulling energy into the body with your intention. Do this for four minutes, breathing energy in from the Earth. Then massage the head to open up that energy area. As you massage the head and neck, you fill the body with energy, bringing it through the legs with your breathing. This opens up those areas of the brain to have conscious contact with the dream field of energy.

Everyone dreams, but you frequently do not remember or bring them back into this world. So, the next step is to program your dreams. Before you go to sleep, say, "I will dream about why my right shoulder is so painful," or "I will dream about how I can release these feelings of sadness inside." You can also write down what it is you wish to do in the dream state. Writing it gives you the visual reading

158

which stimulates the dream network also. And then you must write it down when you recall your dreaming in the morning. Even though you do not understand it right then, you may understand it the next day. It is also good to read or tell your dreams to someone else. Oftentimes, as you tell it or read it, you will get realizations or insights about the symbolism that is involved in the dream.

Using Sound

Soli

Sound and vibration have an effect upon the subconscious mind. They help in centering, especially when the individual is making the sound themselves. It is very much a centering process and allows the energy of the Higher Self to come through. That is its prime focus. Understand, too, my friends, that the subconscious mind is in existence throughout the *whole* body, it is not localized in the brain. In its entirety, there are areas of the brain that might be said to be its localization, but it exists throughout the body, so your whole body has memory. Sound and vibration can work on other areas of the body and, therefore, work on the subconscious mind as well. The body also holds much information from previous lifetimes which came with it when you incarnated into this lifetime. It was implanted within the physical structure of the body and your subconscious. Therefore, sound and vibration can assist in bringing that information forward.

9

Communicating With Your Physical Body

Exercise

Dong How Li

There are some things traditionally in this culture that are hard for you to deal with. The physical is one. Some of you (especially in the New Age movement) find it easy to meditate, be spiritual, and watch your beliefs, and harder to be physical and get the exercise that you need. However, that is what is required to get the energy moving again. Exercise, physical exercise, keeps the energy going. It is necessary for the body. You have heard it said from my part of the world: *before enlightenment, chop wood. Afterwards, chop wood too.*

Diet

Dr. Peebles

It is then for each of you to design your individualized diet. If you are to be healthy and strong, it is for you to find foods that digest, ingest, and assimilate *according to your own system.* If you pay attention to that which supposedly works for others, you are avoiding building a communication system to your own karma, your own environment, your own glands, tissues and organs. Find the diet that works for you.

All of you need the cleansing, so drink plenty of clear fluids such as juices, water, tea, or rice water—anything that keeps the system flushed and attracts all the toxins and moves them out and through the body. Have plenty of vitamins and minerals in your body on a daily basis. Do not wait until you have a symptom. Keep your body energized. Each and every morning, when you awaken, check your body. Find out what it is going to need today so that you are able constantly to prevent attachment to environmental symptoms and illnesses.

I am not overly concerned about the fact that as a nation, your diet is abominable. I am concerned about the fact that so many of you, as individuals, feed into that and allow that diet to manipulate and control you. You should all work on building your individual diets: the foods that work for you, that allow you the energy, that allow you the spiritual vitality. When you have a diet that is adequate, when you eat properly, when you eat foods that are easily digested, ingested, and you still don't have the physical energy, it's high time you woke up and said, "I'm giving myself the energy to be spiritual, but this lack of physical energy is just an experience that I must need."

Certainly you must work on your diet. Don't say it takes too much time and energy and, "Oh, well, I'm living in the United States and each diet is a terrible mess and that's why I'm a mess." No, you *chose* to be in a messed-up dietary system to find out if you have the strength of character to design your own system while living in this confusion, and thereby to become a leader to others.

Certainly, my friends, when you are eating your foods on a daily basis, each and every time you drink anything or eat anything, *bless it in light*. Visualize it nourishing not only your physical body, but your etheric body. Visualize that it's bringing you nutrition, balancing, and cleansing.

Touching

Master Adalfo

There is no substitute for being touched. Touching opens up parts

161

of the body, even though people don't know that it serves them in that way. You go to see a dentist, for example, and his assistant may help you get into the chair. If she or he is good, they may take special care to arrange you nicely in the chair, to touch you, and to open parts of the body which they do not even know they are opening. It is always good to open the heart first, so a person can feel the loving that healing is all about.

Enid

In the United States the word "why" is vitally important to beings. They are always asking, "Why's this happening? What's wrong?" Sometimes there's nothing wrong and to dig for the "why" makes it even worse. Get comfortable with the idea of saying, "Oh, this is an experience. So what I'm going to do is I'm going to allow myself to feel it, and I'm going to lift this experience into a new level of consciousness, into a different level of consciousness and then take a look at this."

When you're not feeling well, it is an experience that is creating an effect upon you. However, if you can just stop for a moment and say, "All right, I don't like this feeling and I want to be feeling better." But do look at what the experience is and *allow yourself to feel it*. Unless you do, it's going to come for you again and again. Say, "All right, I feel this here and this there and this in the other place. I'm really feeling it and I'm going to take some deep breaths now because when I take deep breaths, I can take more." If your shoulder is hurting, you can say, "All right my shoulder, let me see and feel there, just how deep does that hurt go? Oh, way down in there? How interesting." And you just take a look at that and say, "Oh body, I'm just loving you in there so much, are you getting my message?"

If you had a favorite child and it came to you with a terrible pain in the shoulder, you'd touch it and love it and say, "Oh, my darling." You'd kiss it and you'd just take care of it and you'd love it. Well, if you don't do that to your own body, you're missing out on a lot. You need to love your body because it isn't you. It's a *vehicle* for you. It's your own little child and you want to treat it like your own little child and

162

love and caress it. And sometimes if you can't do enough for yourself, you call a friend and say, "You know, I wish you'd rub my shoulder a little bit for me."

You don't have to have someone who is highly trained in healing because healing is endemic to all mankind. It's endemic to all animals. You hold an animal and it heals you; it's a vibration for healing. It's a vibration for love and love is what heals. So you can take advantage of anyone just by asking them to rub your shoulder and ease that pain away for you.

There are some things that you can do when you are all alone. Just caress the body and touch it with loving hands. You know, sometimes when you're not feeling good and that shoulder hurts, you want to chop it off. You want to get away from it. So what you do is you resist that wanting to get away from it and you come close to it. You allow yourself to feel it and be near to it and admit that it's yours. Probably the very best thing that you can do at that point is to take away all judgments like, "What did I do to deserve this? I must have been terrible or something that I deserve this pain." Take away all judgments of what people will think about you if you walk around with this painful shoulder. Take away all judgment about what's happening with the body and understand that this is an experience that you're having. Sometimes an experience can cause us to stop in the middle of the road and look around. We just get on that road and we're going so fast that we never stop to look around. You need to stop and smell the roses sometimes.

So many people think that the world is a dangerous place and they think that the physical Universe is an enemy. "I've got to make it over all of the obstacles here. And I've got to make the physical Universe do what I want it to do, no matter what." But this world wants you to do good; it's just trying its very best to give you everything you want. Sometimes you need to slow down and an illness can do that for you.

Going to the mountains for a couple of days or to the beach can be the best healing in the world. Sometimes, the very best healing is loving yourself enough to take a couple of days off and bring yourself to a beautiful place. Allow things for yourself. We tend to tell ourselves, "You don't deserve this. You can't have that." You wouldn't say that to your favorite child, now would you? You'd say, "You want that? I'll break my back getting it for you." If you'd do that for *yourself*, it would be ever so much better. Do it for you!

Massage

Master Adalfo

Techniques such as massage are valuable, particularly in getting people acquainted with their bodies. In the society in which you live, you sit in chairs, you do not sit on the floor or on the ground. You wear clothes that cover your bodies. You go to doctors and dentists to have things done that people used to take care of themselves. So, you are not acquainted with your bodies; they are almost foreign strangers.

So, massage, acupressure, rolfing, any of these are ways to get more in touch with the *feelings* of your physical body. What we have here is a culture that feels only pain and not pleasure with their physical body. Some of the procedures cause pain at first, and that is all right, because that brings your awareness to that part of the body again and you feel it. Then you can move away from the pain into an enjoyment of that area as the pain goes away, but you still remain aware of that area.

All of these techniques are ways of releasing stress, of releasing toxicity, and also of getting more acquainted with the body and knowing where the problem areas are *before* they have to become a terrible disease to make you aware of them. If you feel a little bit of a pinch when someone is massaging you, that is better than having to have surgery in that area so you'd *really* feel it.

Laying-On-Of-Hands Healing

Soli

What, then, of apparently miraculous healings, laying-on-of-hands, and energy transference? Of course, they are real. But there are no such things as what you call "miracles." Everything is a

164

miracle (or not a miracle, depending on your point of view). There is no one thing that is any more miraculous than another. Everyone has the power of energy transference. You can all transfer power from your Higher Self through your hands to another individual. It is up to the individual and his or her Higher Self whether that energy is utilized or not, as to whether you have effectively healed that person or not.

What, then, of the effective healers? What, then, of the large numbers who appear to be healed? First, ask yourself, "Why are those individuals there? Why are they with those diseases seeking to be cured? What of those who are cured?" It is because those individuals have a need for something within their lives to draw them out of the subconscious belief patterns that they have held onto so strongly for so long. A healing, an apparently miraculous healing, is something totally unexpected for them, something totally outside of their immediate awareness, totally outside of anything that they have dealt with before in their life to that date. It has a tremendous impact upon the subconscious mind and its belief systems. It blows wide open all the limiting beliefs that they have held onto so tightly for so long.

There are some individuals who require the experience of a miraculous healing upon the Earth plane. Their Higher Selves wish them to have that sudden opening, sudden awareness, sudden expansion of their belief system into a totally new area. So, the Higher Self creates the circumstances in which they will receive that energy, where they will receive an apparent healing. It does, in many cases, transform the individual's life. Generally speaking, it is those individuals who have dealt with a very dogmatic, very closed belief system for a long time. Such so-called "faith healing" works far less effectively on those individuals who are already upon the path to enlightenment and self-awareness. Why is this? Because those individuals already *know* they are responsible for their own lives, that they must take responsibility for the creation of the disease. Since they take responsibility for the creation of the disease, they equally take responsibility for its disbursement, its alleviation.

Master Adalfo

To make the laying-on-of-hands healing more effective means to be more loving, and loving comes in all guises. Loving does not mean unconditional support for any kind of behavior. That is not loving, that is destroying.

If you are a healer, when you care about a client and bring the caring to the client through your hands, that enhances the value of laying-on-of-hands healing. But part of your intent must be to love the client, to care for the client, not just, "This is a way of passing half an hour of my day," but a commitment of caring, a commitment of nurturing, a commitment of loving. If there is someone that you cannot love in any way, you should please send them to someone else. They should not be your client because how will they get well when healing does not include loving? It is important always to remember that healing is loving and loving is healing, for without that, it cannot take place.

Lessons From Nature

Ting-Lao

Laying-on-of-the-hands healing can do much for the auto-immune system. It is very effective, in fact, for killing the virus also. It is easy to kill a virus. All you need to do is do it. It is only a bug in the body and like any other virus, it can be radiated with the energy which is amplified through the body and hands. This is very effective. Those in the fields of healing should study the immune systems of animals more, in terms of their energy fields. See what happens energy-wise. They do have ways of healing themselves, you know, with mud and fasting. People do know of these ways, but they have not studied the actual auto-immune system of animals enough. I know it is a sacrifice for the animals to be used in laboratory research, but again, they come to *serve* in this way. Study them in an energy way, with clairvoyants and psychics to read the energies of the animals.

166

You can learn much about how to train the energies of the ill person to fight in proper ways, so that they won't wear out the system, or wear down the system, or exhaust the system, thus disabling it to fight when it is needed. It would be good, if people could study the patterns, energy-wise, in the birds. I know it sounds odd, but birds are very wise beings. Mammals are usually used in medical research because they are similar anatomically to people. But you who know of energy ways could do well to study birds because their bodies are very fine, very delicate, very finely tuned and coordinated. So, if you studied the intricate energies of the birds, it will help you to be aware of the intricate energy systems in the mammals and humans, and to get out of that mode of just dealing with the physical level of the auto-immune system.

10

Traditional Healing

Cures/Vaccines

Soli

When it is no longer necessary to have a disease such as AIDS upon the Earth plane, when no one needs that experience anymore, then someone from the Spirit side may very well pass the idea to someone on the Earth plane and a so-called "cure" will come forward. But there will always be some other illness waiting in the wings, some other way to exit for the human being who is choosing to leave the Earth plane. *Cures come when the disease is no longer necessary.* There are no accidents. As long as there are those who need to have the experience of leaving the Earth by AIDS or have the need for the experience of the communication of AIDS (and changing their lives because of it), it will stay upon the Earth plane. Always. Those within the Spirit dimension will not interfere in *any way* with the Earth plane. It is always the choice of those on the Earth as to their needs and their path.

As more and more individuals go within and discover their own inner guidance, work on themselves, take responsibility for their own lives, then less and less is their need for what some would see as catastrophe or tragedy. There will be those who chose to leave through Earth changes, volcanic eruptions, airplane crashes, all forms of departure. And when there is no further need for those experiences, then there will be no further need for that illness or experience to be manifest and it will go away.

Zoosh

An outgrowth of the medical and chemical research will be a mass vaccination in the form of a serum that will "cure" AIDS. With this research, a sudden realization will arise as to how many diseases can be cured through the use of a chemically-induced genetic change within the body. It will be very close to involving the human being on an *emotional level* to create genetic change, using the chemical as a catalyst to bring about that change. So, really, this is another step towards discontinuing a disease through the use of your emotional, mental, spiritual and physical processes alone, without the help of a chemical inducer.

This vaccination and the immunological treatment and research will bring about the cure of many diseases. Part of that treatment will promote people to change their attitudes as well. The research going on now will tend to support that within a three to five year period. It will also be possible, before too long, with the use of chemical and emotional changes, to change the body genetically in such a way that the immune system does not ever contract disease. This is all possible within your lifetimes.

Dong How Li

Now, curiously, a vaccine will be one more invasion. It is designed to boost the immune system but it will be an invasion again. The danger here is that those who receive this new invasion will think they have developed their immune systems to fight for themselves, when really, some of these vaccines *will not* be doing that. Some of the vaccines will be replacing their own immune systems instead of helping their immune systems to be more vital.

Now, this is only the physical layer of it. What is going on subconsciously and on the symbolic level is more important: namely, by accepting a vaccine of that nature and thereby getting strong enough to fight, you are still not fighting your battle with your own strength. You are taking someone else's issues and using them to stand on. That will work for a time until the next battle rages and you find you still don't have your own feet to stand on. This is why it is so important for you to read this material on AIDS because nowhere else is anyone approaching this from so many perspectives and making them available for getting underneath, above, or around the obvious.

Doctors

Dr. Peebles

My friends, recognize that if you are to maintain your physical health, it is important to build an attitude within your own conscious mind, an attitude of acknowledgment and of acceptance of the fact that healing is individualized, *that healing is something that you do not create, but that you allow.* In a way, that is creation; it is a creation of the Loving Law of Allowance. For instance, suppose you do not believe in the medical profession, you do not believe in doctors, and you also tell people around you, "Oh, I don't believe in doctors. You shouldn't go to a doctor. You can do it this way. You can do it that way." Then you are contributing to interference for them and for yourself. There are many who *should* go to the doctor for the doctors are (in fact) guided by the Spirit. Doctors also are *guided* by the Universal God or they would not have studied to learn how to heal. Yes, they too are healers. If you, then, have put that mistrust of doctors into motion in your mind, eventually you will have the need for a doctor. If you then turn to the doctor and say, "Oh well, I didn't believe and I don't believe in doctors, but in this particular case it's my problem, my health, so I'm coming to the doctor anyway," then you will not be healed, no matter how close to healing your soul is. Because of what you have put into motion, the healing will not work. The doctor will not be able to define it, and will not be able to find what will actually work for you because your aura, your consciousness has already spent a great deal of time rejecting it. And so, you will have deluded yourself and you have created the opportunity for spiritual disillusionment.

170

Master Adalfo

One of the goals that we have for the Aquarian Age would be the coming together of the esoteric knowledge and the esoteric, which is public knowledge.

There are several ways. We must have more doctors that are more open. Healers who use methods of healing that are outside the orthodox mode must first be willing to accept those in the medical profession on their level and then exchange ideas with them. We can never expect doctors to be less cynical of alternative healing methods if we are overly cynical of what they do. Why should the burden be all on them and not on those of you who do these other kinds of healing? You must be able to accept the good work that medical doctors do. Encourage people, when that is important for them, to see a medical doctor. If you are a healer, perhaps you could talk to that person's doctor. Ask questions. Do you know the method of using inquiry? Ask the doctor questions because you care about this client and because you want to know.

And you can say, "Yes, I can see how that will help me as I work with this client." The doctor may then ask you questions. Do not be defensive in your answers; just be direct and explain what it is you are doing. And if the doctor says, "That is foolish. That will never work," then say, "I understand that you see it that way." And because you do understand that, you understand his limitations. And that understanding is what is required.

Understanding also requires that healers become more aware of scientific language so that they can actually discuss something with the doctor and not expect him to learn their language. So, it requires giving on both sides. We do see more and more doctors taking a healing class here and there, nurses also. And as more of that happens, we will see more of an exchange.

171

Understanding Viruses

Ting-Lao

We want to say a little bit about viruses in general, and about the AIDS virus which is one of them. Those in the field of medicine know how viruses mutate, or that they do mutate, and know that they cannot be killed. We want to address this on the energy level, or the spiritual level, because it is important now for medicine to be entertaining the possibility of the *consciousness* of the virus. This is the *only* way that medicine is going to be able to conquer it. The virus has a will of its own. It multiplies and has a purpose. The people whom it infects do not have as much of an awareness of their own will or sense of purpose as the virus does. The virus has one thing in mind and that is to do all of the things that it does.

So, we would like to suggest to the medical community and scientific community that they talk philosophically about the enti-tyness of the virus. They should observe the patterns and the personalities of the people that the virus infects, or affects, and see the relationships there. By treating the virus as an entity, it would help to knock it off its feet and to knock its knees out from underneath it. It needs to be attacked from this angle. The scientific and medical community is attacking it from the physical level with drugs and all these kinds of things, but it is very difficult to succeed because the virus gets used to the drugs just as the insects get used to pesticides. The virus needs to be attacked on the non-physical planes, dimensions, or realms. This has to do with getting inside of the virus's thought processes–inside their purpose for being. People need to be less oblivious to this aspect of working with viruses.

When Drugs Work Or Don't Work

Soli

Any drug, any external chemical that is put into the physical body in order to cure a symptom is going to cause its own problems.

172

Understand that a *physical symptom within the body is ultimately the outer symptom of the inner disease*. The drugs are aimed at curing the symptom, and until the underlying disease is dealt with, there can be no cure. The drugs might alleviate the symptom for a time, but that is all they will do. The danger for society is that it is placing so much emphasis on drugs, believing the mechanical cure is the only cure possible, and the only cure necessary. So individuals will be searching for a mechanical cure, instead of understanding its underlying creation is in the psyche.

The drugs will never work. They will cure the symptoms for a time and life will be prolonged temporarily. They have value from that point of view, to gain time for the individual to work on self, to begin to change the belief systems of the subconscious, to begin to turn around feelings about self and how they view themselves and life. Many, of course, will not do so even then, for they have such total belief in the mechanical model of illness that they will expect the drugs to cure them completely. And, after all, look at the energy in society at this time. People are blaming the government for not having spent billions of dollars to find the AIDS cure already. Everyone is looking in the wrong direction. The mechanical cure will be found accidently one day when the underlying disease has been dealt with in your society. Then, that mechanical drug will assist the physical body to recuperate without creating more problems than it solves.

All the drugs that you are dealing with right now have side effects and they create their own problems within the physical. You are simply shifting the symptom from one area of the physical body into another area of the physical body, where it might not even manifest for months or years. But, it has value and is positive in the sense that the individuals taking drugs believe in them, and their subconscious believes and, thus, it allows a certain healing to take place. It buys time for individuals to work on self and understand what physical disease is.

Safe Sex

Soli

Because there is such a fear out there, because there is that particular energy of this AIDS mechanism, it has its own power. Each is involved in the collective unconscious. If you rebel against a moral code, if you rebel against the collective unconscious belief system, then you are not going to transcend it, you will be *caught up* in the webs of that belief system. What we are suggesting is that individuals need, ultimately, to go within and free themselves from this collective belief system and find their own internal reality and belief, and transcend that.

However, we understand that most people are not in that position, and because the belief in a mechanical distribution of this illness is so powerful and strong, most will believe in it. So, it is important that they follow the beliefs about the mechanics of it. If people continue to have sex, then it is important that they follow those practices of contraception because their minds are going to be telling them that if they don't, they will catch this disease. It is necessary to work with the belief systems of the mind as they exist at the moment. If you believe, "I will catch this disease if I don't do this, that, and the other thing," then you'd better do this, that, and the other thing until such a time as you can go beyond the belief and transcend it. While the belief is there, while individuals are so caught up in the belief system of society, follow the suggestions of "safe sex."

11

Non-Traditional Healing

Ting-Lao

One should go inside the consciousness of the virus, just as you meld with a lover when you are making love, or just as Mr. Spock does mind-meld. Go inside the other and know what they know, feel what they feel, and think what they think. Let yourself meld. Do not fear that the virus will eat you up because if you fear it, that gives it fuel, food. But if you do not fear this, then you can keep your will intact and withdraw yourself. So, yes, one should attack viruses from that level. Just talk to it like any other beingness by saying, "What are you doing here? What are you all about?" Then tell it to leave and harness your will. You have more will than it has, and the greater will wins.

Basically, all healing methods are the same in most cultures. It is the words, ideas, and concepts that are different. They are the same in the aspect that they use energy to heal and to open up the body, or to close down parts of it. This regulates the flow of the energy, closing down the parts that may be leaking or losing energy and opening up the parts that are not drawing in enough energy such as a pancreas or a heart. So it is all a matter of modulating and regulating the energy flow so that each cell in the body can have the energy that it needs. There is no one way that is perfect, no one way that is right while other ways are not so right. Every way is different and has its own advantages and disadvantages.

There is acupuncture, massage, yoga, the Shaman ways of chant-

ing, dancing, ceremonies, laying-on-of-hands healing, and psycho-
therapeutic counseling. There are very many ways of healing. All of
them use energy and also retrack and retrain the flow of energy
through the body. They all complement each other and can work
together. So I am saying that even though the healing methods are
different, they all have one similar goal and that is to *retrain* the
energy flow through the body or mind.

Group Work

Ting-Lao

One must accept one's friends and relatives with unconditional
love. Many people who have AIDS feel that they are doing this now,
and by doing so, they feel loved themselves on a deeper level. It is like
needing to reparent each other. In this situation, *conditional* love
also takes place. This is like a stern parent who watches and guides
what his or her child does in order to help. The parent says, "I don't
think what you are doing is good for you. You need to change, and do
such and such." This is a kind of helping, but it is also a conditional
love.

Group fellowship can help the members of the group grow and
change through unconditional love, a very special and deep love, love
on its highest level. Many people resent being reparented because of
their own poor parenting. Our job is to move on from that as we
reparent each other into greater happiness. Remember, all parents
do what they do, and they do their best.

We are all here to enjoy life fully. However, we need to confront
each other occasionally and say that what the other person is doing
is not good for his enjoyment of life. This gives one a feeling of deep
caring, while actually helping the person.

I think it is quite helpful to form a group and work together. You
can have a leader, but it is not necessary. It is important to really
work at loving each other, hugging each other, listening and paying
attention to each other. You open up and express your feelings and
understand how you need to bring some changes into your lives. It is

a bit like group therapy. I feel that people truly care for each other when they band together like this. In such a group, you need to give each other strong support and encouragement. You might say, "You need to do this. This is your goal for next week. What are you going to do about it? We will see you next week." Yes, you need to set goals for yourselves, then when you get together you can compare notes. This can be done with gentle suggestions or a polite kick in the rear with your spiritual boots. You need to energize yourselves so that changes can be made to get rid of this illness.

So, how do we deal with a friend who has this illness? It is difficult to trust their process because, obviously, there is something awry which caused the illness in the first place. It is also difficult to trust one's own process if you, too, hold these same doubts and fears. The key may lie within group therapy. Just sitting together creates more energy, but you must be watchful that it doesn't become fearful energy. Fears can feed each other. But, group togetherness can help to overcome those tendencies. Healthy vibrations can be emphasized and indeed created through group sittings, which will enable you to overcome the suppressed anger and self-esteem, emotions often ignored since childhood.

Don't coddle those that are in their sickness, you see. They need to get on the ball, otherwise they are not going to be able to make the necessary changes to rid themselves of this illness. The reason for telling someone that you do not feel it is such a bright idea for them to be doing something is because there's not enough light in that situation for their progress. You are speaking to them out of love.

In metaphysical circles, some believe that giving joy and pure, unconditional love is enough to cure illness. However, even if pure, unconditional love were given to someone steadily, even if you poured a constant flow upon him, and cared for him and did things without expectations, this may still not help. What he may need to hear is, "You need to call your mother and tell her how you really feel about her." Something difficult like that.

Groups are good, but they may have grave failings in their attempts to heal, that they do not treat the person on enough energy levels. The person often thinks that attending the group is all he

177

needs to do. They do not expand themselves enough to encompass all the therapies and all the levels of complexities of this disease and of life. People, in general, take life too simplistically and try to understand human nature and themselves too simplistically, and so they try to deal with this disease in too simplistic a way. Also, they depend too much on others and do not do enough themselves.

The group therapies need to be much tougher about shaking and waking and breaking up these patterns in their people. They need to say, "You need to look at what you must change in your life and how you are going to get better. You know, you are not well now. This is an indication of imbalance. What you need to do is to bring yourself back into balance." Each group has its idea of what the members need to do: either to love themselves or take care of things within their families, or to just express love. There are many different ways of helping and all people have what *they think* is the answer. What they need to do is to *combine* everybody's answer and share, and not be competitive and not think that any one way is right because no one way is right for everyone. Most people need ten therapies and ten ways: not specifically ten, but much more than they are getting.

The Power Of Will

Ting-Lao

The primary defense against AIDS is physical. It is a physical disease and the virus is a physical entity. So, the primary defenses are physical, avoiding those things which are known to be able to infect you. In addition to that, physically one can work with one's *will* ahead of time on preventative health. The will is like an energy essence living in the body, in the lower abdomen, and it is that force that people can use. It is that force that mothers use to lift cars off their children in an accident. It is that sheer power that you hear about in stories of that kind.

In American society, one does not have much will, because from childhood people are told what to do, instead of being educated and trained to think, feel and interact in a communicating way with one's

178

own feelings and thoughts, as well as those of others. Therefore, the will gets put aside.

However, everyone can train their children to participate in constructive projects that teach them about the energy world and teach them about manifesting what they want and need by harnessing their will and giving it the *power of the word*. You have often heard that the word creates, just as it says in the Bible and in many other metaphysical texts. The word is power and thought is power. Oftentimes, word and thought only stay on the auditory or mental plane. It must be harnessed with will from the actual body in order to manifest into the physical-life plane. People can begin to use *their* will as preventative health maintenance. In this way, people can train their children to use their will. So, this is a psychic way to help one defend oneself, *not in place of* the physical, but *in addition to* the physical precautions.

Now, of course, to be on one's spiritual path is important. It means to be more aware. The price of being on one's path is to pay attention. Paying attention is the price for knowing your way or being able to find your guidance. You have to pay attention to your physical body and the feelings there. You have to pay attention to your emotional body and the feelings there. You have to pay attention to your mental programmings and thoughts. You have to pay attention to guidance, whether from God or Spirit Guides or from philosophy. All these things need one's attention and awareness. This is the meaning of being conscious: *you are conscious of what is going on.* Being spiritually healthy will help one to be strong when this virus is multiplying and multiplying throughout the society.

179

VII

Helping

"*Understand that the being who agrees to such an experience of AIDS is exceedingly brave and must be treated as such. All beings are not willing to experience it. A lot of the experience of AIDS has to do with others viewing the courage. . . .There are beings here on this planet who don't want to live with ordinary feelings and an ordinary way of life. They need to have a deep and profound experience in order to grow spiritually and they have planned for that experience. . . .Those who have the deepest experiences become the most courageous people on the planet.*"

1

If You Are Experiencing AIDS

Enid

My darling, I'm very proud of you because, if you're suffering from AIDS, it means that you have a deep willingness to experience life at its deepest, most important and significant levels. Sometimes that can be very small comfort when you're feeling terrible within yourself; you feel almost deathfulness within you. But understand that isn't *death* that you're feeling, but *new life*. And, in order to have the new life that you've ordered for yourself (before you took on your body), you must have some deep experience that will drive you into newness of thought, newness of awareness and understanding. Those friends of yours who also are suffering from AIDS, you'll see those levels of courage behind their eyes that you never noticed were there before. If you look very hard and strong into the mirror, you'll see it in yourself.

Understand that life on this plane is lived on different levels. For instance, there is a higher part of you that is applauding your experience, applauding you for the willingness to dig deep into the physical experience. All beings who come here do so for the expressed purpose of expanding their experience so that when they go back to life as Spirits, they have wonderful richness with which to feel themselves expanded. Any experience that you've had in your life forever changes your view of yourself and your view of life. That's what you take with you when you leave the body. You really *can* take it with you. You take all the richness of experience, all the greater depth of understanding.

Also understand that you live a *snowflake* kind of existence, which is different from any other. Just as your fingerprints are different from all others, your uniqueness is a mark of your separateness and your ability to experience separation. However, all of life's experiences are later shared with all other beings in existence because *we are all one.* Your experience, whether you realize it or not, is shared with *all* other life. All other life will gain by the depth of this experience. You may feel like there is nothing wonderful about pain, there is nothing wonderful about devastation of the body. I know how you feel in what you're experiencing right now.

Know that if this experience were not real for you, and if it weren't felt with great depth, you would never gain what you wanted to gain by it. In order to experience this at all, you have been masterful in creating a state of reality for yourself in which it could happen. So you must applaud yourself instead of judging yourself harshly. It's very easy to judge oneself harshly when you are suffering and you feel totally inept and totally useless as far as being able to cause change.

Oh, but darling, you're not useless, and it's not hopeless. In order for us to come through to greater understanding on any subject, on any plane of existence, we must first stretch the membranes of our minds and hearts and awareness. That's what you are doing now, as terrible as it might seem. For you, because of your great depth of beingness, your experience had to be exceedingly dire. It had to be exceedingly great for you to garner the energy that was necessary to create states of mind that you have wanted to experience. These are states of mind that will help catapult you into enormous understanding, enormous awareness—the states of mind that are necessary for you to create in order to experience further worlds that you have planned for your future.

You see, as hard as this world is, as difficult as it is to understand, there are even more difficult worlds, and for some of you (not for all) it is important that you stretch yourself to your outermost possible limits in order to prepare for these other worlds. Now you might say, "Well, that's easy for you to say, you're not lying here suffering the way I am. You haven't seen the devastation. You haven't felt the deep terror, the betrayal that I feel. I feel the world has betrayed me." But understand, my darling, it's a *part of the experience that you created.*

You may totally disagree with my words. They may not comfort you on the surface. But beneath that surface (where there is greater understanding) you are responding, and these vibrations will help you with the healing of your mind. It is the *healing of the mind* that is taking place in this dreadful illness of the body.

If you can, just hold those words close to your heart for a few moments, and know there is great truth in them. Whether you can totally understand it or not, allow the words to give you comfort because *we all love you.* All your Spirit Guides are applauding you. They're cheering you on. And you must know that although you may feel shunned and looked down upon, there are those who are jealous of your courage. Deep down, they're thinking, "Oh, how could I ever have experienced this?"

The important thing is that you persist and gather as much of the energy of this experience as you can to cause a metamorphosis in your heart, mind, and understanding. It takes great energy to create these levels of consciousness. There are so many different levels of consciousness and those which you seek take great depths in order to reach them. Remember about the great energies. Put these into a great big ball and help them shove you through the window of your understanding.

The moment you can allow energy to work for you, even your body will ease and you will begin to feel better. So use that energy. It's true for any experience. We can use these great, strong energies to literally propel ourselves through to new understanding. The only things that really and truly happen are those within the self–deep inside, inside your heart. You're experiencing this on many levels. On other levels, for those who view you, you're raising their consciousness regarding feelings of compassion and understanding.

Now don't forget to love yourself. A part of this gathering of experience and coming up through to greater understanding is gaining understanding and love of yourself, and learning not to judge yourself. Know how brave you are, how beautiful, and how wonderful.

185

This disease does not describe you. It is only an experience—only that.

I want to thank you for being willing to discover the depths of experience on this plane of existence. I love you very much, and I'm always there. You can call upon me, Enid, at any time. Just say, "Oh Enid, please come and talk with me," and I'll be there for you.

You Are An Example Of Courage

Jesus of the Light

Understand, my dear ones, if you are experiencing AIDS, then you have chosen to show yourselves a communication in a way that is very uncomfortable for you, and you can, if you choose, end your lives here, and thereby end your denial of who you really are, or you can choose to live in the most healthy way that you have ever lived. I am not suggesting that you give up or deny yourself any experience, but rather, that you stop using the experience of AIDS as a defense.

Recognize that because you are who you are, you have the stigmatic effect of AIDS. That is how the world that you live in perceives it at this time, as being a stigma. You know this and it is not unusual for you to feel rejected, abandoned and, in some cases, even defensive or aggressive. It is not because you are different, or that you are less of a person, or that you are more of one; it is that your world has set up an artificial standard of what is health, of what is strength, of what is beauty, and so on. It is for you, if you would, to accept your leadership role of establishing a different way of being.

Do not attack those who are not like you by saying, "I am right in my way of life and you are wrong." And do not feel that you must defend yourself to those who say, "You are wrong and are being punished." Rather say to those who attack you, "I am a child of God. I am a child of light. I am a speaker of my own truth. I am a speaker of light. You may or may not choose to believe I am who I am. I choose to believe it and that is enough. I make no apology for who I am, nor do I demand apologies from you. I am that I am and that is enough for me."

If you are willing, my friends, to say this for yourself and for

186

others, you will fulfill all obligations of the election of you, by you, to have this disease. It is only that–an election. You have volunteered in many ways, in your soul self, to expose the world to alternate realities, alternate ways of living; you have chosen to participate in the group of those who live alternately, by experiencing the stigma that has been applied to them by the world in general.

For those of you who participate in this experience, understand that you have, on a soul level, volunteered and you have, on a soul level, been elected. On the God level and on the light level, you have been greatly appreciated for your actions. And a few of you may thank yourself and excuse yourself from a continuation of the experience.

Taulmus

To those souls who have manifested this disease, AIDS, and who are seeing, on a deeper level, the results and effects of this sickness in their bodies and in their lives, I wish to offer commendation for their courage and steadfastness through a most difficult and agonizing time of siege. These individuals are demonstrating what, in truth, is a malady that is not their responsibility alone, but belongs to the entire body of humanity. AIDS is simply the effect of the *collective unconscious* of all who dwell in your physical world. These souls of which I speak have done a great service for their fellow humans and should be given the support and empathy due them, rather than the discrimination and ostracizing that is taking place in many circles against them.

Examples Of Courage In Others

Dong How Li

We can all learn from examples of courage and initiation like Rock Hudson. Do you know that when you have courage, you take one or two steps forward, then you panic and pull back? He did the same thing. He committed to this path before he arrived in the body. It was a major act of initiation for him to expose himself publicly. He did,

187

after all, have a choice. He chose consciously, to expose himself publicly. It is true that eventually other people would have found out by rumor, but he chose to announce it to the media himself. In the moment of his courage, he was a hero. Afterwards, in the moment of his fear, he was a victim. He went back and forth, even as each of you do at every initiation level.

Disease, in itself, doesn't make you a hero. The situation doesn't make you a hero. *How you approach it* is what makes you a hero. You must approach it with compassion and without recklessness and with some larger cause in mind other than your own well being. For a culture that worships heroes, it is amazing to us that you have so few today.

You will notice that there are people in this culture now who are not in the media forefront, not on the front page, but who are taking stands for their gay brothers and sisters. There are people who are frightened themselves but are trying to help, perhaps shaking in their boots, but these are the seeds of your new heroism. You must take it upon yourselves to honor each other because the media will not do so. Please extend that honor to include the doctors, who, in their own fields, are as stymied as you are, and are heroically seeking something indefinable.

Enid

Understand that the being who agrees to such an experience of AIDS is exceedingly brave and must be treated as such. All beings are not willing to experience it. A lot of the experience of AIDS has to do with others viewing the courage of those affected. If you will notice, many of the beings who have AIDS speak with great courage. You find yourself very moved by that. You don't find them kicking and screaming and feeling sorry for themselves.

For example, look at Rock Hudson. That was the way he wanted to go out, sort of in a blaze of glory, having done something for others. He agreed to go public, also. He could have stayed private. He had a very hard time with it, but he had to follow through. Seeing someone of his stature suffer in this way brought out the compassion in people.

188

Because he was so loved and adored worldwide for his films, because people cared and loved him so much, when they saw him suffer, they didn't care that he was homosexual. He was able to bring out compassion that otherwise would not have been brought out.

There are beings here on this planet who don't want to live with ordinary feelings and an ordinary way of life. They need to have a deep and profound experience in order to grow spiritually and they have planned for that experience. Those who are in need of that experience are saying, "I'm coming into awakening, and I still have not had the rough and deep experience I planned for. Where is it?" And here comes AIDS.

Can you understand how all this is serving mankind in many wonderful ways? Those who have the *deepest experiences* are the most courageous ones on the planet. They have been able to make the world real to that degree, through this disease, and that is very hard to do. You know that is so, once you have awakened. You know how hard it is to make certain things real to yourself because you've already seen the sky.

The courage of those with AIDS serves as an inspiration for others, and we wonder if we would be able to be like that, to have that courage, if we were experiencing the disease ourselves. But you have experienced this already because they are mirroring your courage, your feelings of compassion and love. They are incredible mirrors, just as the sweet little babies in Africa and India who are starving are wonderful mirrors for us, mirrors of *willingness to experience life as it comes.*

Dr. Peebles

Some of you may remember the story of Miriam in the Christian Bible. Miriam was a paraplegic. She was able to physically mature, but she was still a paraplegic and was most miserable. Her personality was critical of herself and everyone. She was called what would be a "shrew."

Her father, hearing that the teacher Jesus was passing through the village, went to him and said, "I am a wealthy man. You and your followers are welcome to stay in my home. Those who cannot fit in my home are welcome to camp on my grounds. I will feed you and clothe you if you will heal my daughter."

So Jesus went to see the girl. He spoke to her, saying, "My dear, I am able to heal your soul, but I am unable to heal your body." She became enraged and screamed and cried and carried on. And so the father would not allow them to stay, for he could not accept that her body could not be healed.

Many, many months went by. Jesus returned and said once more, "I am able to heal your soul, but I cannot heal your body." For you see, hers was not a body experience. It was not a consciousness experience of free will. It was her karma, her need, to have that physical body. And so, in frustration, she gave in and Jesus was able to meditate, pray and heal her soul.

From that point on, she was never depressed or angry again. People would come from miles around and Miriam would sing to them, sing to them the songs of faith, sing to them the songs of encouragement. She would tell them stories of communication, telepathically, emotionally, spiritually. She spent the rest of her life as a worker for the great teacher Jesus, but as a paraplegic.

And so it is that you with AIDS must look and see. There are many souls who come into bodies never to have the need for illness, but get caught up so much in the fears that they manifest it. They can soul-heal themselves. Sometimes you are able to work with them and their souls will be healed; the illness will be in remission and healing. There are some that you could do everything for and nothing will work, for they came into that body to have that experience, which for them it is a soul experience.

2

If Your Loved Ones Are Experiencing AIDS

Sharing The Experience

Jesus of the Light

For those of you who have a loved one who is experiencing AIDS, understand that it is not designed for you to suffer, or to feel as though you are being left out. For, indeed, in many ways you will feel as though you have been stigmatized by association, and feel guilty, to some extent, from the reactions of others. You may feel guilty for not having that same disease which your friends or family members have.

Realize that your purpose is not to have that experience at this time, but to *witness* it, for in the witnessing you will find a great sense of freedom and expressiveness flowing within you. You will have a desire to create a freer and more lasting peace within yourself, a peace that is designed for your own joy, for your own harmony. By doing this, you will also promote joy and harmony in others and help them to see themselves as individual beings in the light of God, as individual soul lights in the great energy of God.

To help them to see themselves as empowered beings in their own right, you do not need to believe that any disease can be caught from them or that any disease would be necessarily attracted to you by merely being exposed to those individuals that you know and cherish. It is rather for you to share the experiences of your loved ones in their final days, or share in their cures, should they cure themselves. It is possible.

Keep a notebook of your own feelings, and record what comes up when you are alone with your friends and dear ones and what you are thinking about and talking about with others. Do this for yourselves, primarily as a gift to yourself and as a reminder of your experience with your dear ones. For those of you who feel so inspired, after the departure of your dear ones or after their healings, keep the notebook or diary and be willing to write about it and share portions of it with others. Do not expect it to become a best-seller; rather treasure it as notes to yourself about your dear ones.

Understand that it is very important for people to hear from someone whom they feel is an observer, someone who is removed in the way that a journalist, a reporter, a witness is, as to what this is all about. You are all human beings. And there is always a big interest in who you are and in what you can do for each other and what you feel for each other. You can have the greatest effect on others in your lives if you are willing to be a good witness, a good friend, a good companion, and to extend that companionship to others, even though they may not understand your experience as a witness or your dear one's experience as one who lives with the disease AIDS.

Understand that you will have the experience of anger from time to time. You also will have the experience of forgiveness for yourself. And you will have that anger and forgiveness of the anger of those who do not understand. You will experience forgiveness for the anger of those who participate in the disease and for others who witness it.

Forgiveness is the experience that will release the bondage from this disease, as well as from all diseases. It is the anger which is not heard from that brings forth disease in general. It is those variations and differing forms of anger which are unheard, unexpressed, and judged which bring forth disease.

You, my friends, as witnesses, can do a great deal to spread the word of education and love for those who experience, for those who witness, for those who observe, as well as for those who judge this disease. It is through friendliness, love, appreciation, acceptance, and forgiveness that this disease and all diseases will be *re-estab-*

192

lished in harmony in the physical self. This disease will not be conquered. If it is conquered, then it will again be Armageddon.

If it is loved into re-energizing somewhere else as comfort, harmony, self-love, friendship, joy, awakening, light, this disease can be a gift in disguise. Yes, a gift in disguise! For that which points out a discomfort in you and a discomfort in society as a whole can truly be a friend in disguise.

My friends, my dear ones, all of you, be open to the possibility of *growing through* disease by *growing past* disease, by *growing into harmony* in all ways: with each other, with yourself, and with your world or Universe. Forgive yourself and all others for all true misdeeds as well as for misdeeds that have been imagined. The key to health and harmony is forgiveness as well as tolerance. Tolerance is an aspect of forgiveness, but forgiveness is the personalization of love.

Giving Love And Respect

Dr. Peebles

If you want to help, you must say that AIDS is *not* an abomination. AIDS is not a curse for what you did wrong, thought wrong, or said wrong. AIDS is little more than another illness that is sweeping the world. We have to combat it with our love and respect, using whatever possible tools that are available to give each and every patient, each and every member of each patient's family, the ability to love, to accept each other. Treat the patient as if they had cancer, or a broken bone. Treat them with as much love as you can give.

Work for the protection of human consciousness, human free will, human rights. Stand up for the equality of all living things: animal, plants, and humans. Be gentle but firm demonstrators of peace, light, and truth. Carry the spiritual responsibility of making safe environments. If someone is ill, invite them in. If someone is in need, help them. If a stranger has the same need as your very dear friend, help them equally. Do not impose your help upon another, but be *available* to them.

193

Zoosh

Those of you who are either left behind or are considering that this might take place in the future, be *proud of your loved ones*. Know that they are involved in a great demonstration for mankind, even though your planet has now experienced this both negatively and positively. It has experienced this positively in the sense that it is showing that love between individuals is all right, which has not been really heard and understood before. Your loved ones have chosen to demonstrate that just by loving another person of their choice they have become ill. This has always been the lesson of all your "so-called" social diseases. The equal and opposite reaction to that lesson is also true. Loving an individual of your choice can be through health. That is the lesson of all "so-called" social diseases: love is its own truth.

Understand that for those of you who are left behind or are living with those who are experiencing that disease, I cannot tell you that your loved ones will be with you at all. Some of them may be if they can work on changing their attitudes, and flying in the face of their circumstances, remain cheerful. This is the attitudinal change which is required: to be positive, to not experience negative reality on an emotional level.

Be Gentle With Yourself

Master Adalfo

The AIDS experience is very hard on you. It is very sad and it is very scary. All of those things are true. You need to be very *gentle* with yourself. You must understand that you need to look at your feelings, your fear, your resentment that someone you love is choosing to leave in this way.

You are angry also. You are angry because you are being deserted. That is what you are feeling. If you can let some of those feelings out in an acceptable way, like writing them down, throwing away a few pieces of change in the woods (as a giveaway), then you can begin to approach one another in the family and talk about your feelings. You

194

need, most of all, to love one another. You also need desperately to *touch one another*. At a time when people are afraid of touching, that is when you need it most.

I have said before that healing is touching and touching is healing. This is true for dealing with your feelings also. You need to touch yourself, to feel your own body. You need to touch one another, to hold one another at a time when you are very sad. If you know someone whose loved one has this disease, you need to hold them so they know they aren't alone. Touching is what tells them, "I am not separate. I am a part of the whole Universe because here is someone else touching me." We react so strongly to the tactile and this is very important. So, touch and hold one another so you can feel the union and know that you are not separate. It is that terrible feeling of separation which feels like the tearing of a piece of fabric.

Remember that death is the *beginning of another journey*. It is not the end. And when someone goes on a journey, there are many ways of communicating. We can send postcards, we can write letters, we have the telephone. People forget that you can use those same ways to communicate to those who are on another plane of existence. There is no reason why you cannot write a letter to someone who has passed. Put it under your pillow and invite them to answer it in a dream. Invite them to phone you and make time in your life to sit, so you can take the phone call, so you can *hear them, feel them* near you.

Ask someone else to read the letter, to communicate with them, someone like a medium, someone who can be in between the worlds. This does not have to be a direct voice medium who brings in your loved one to talk to you, but one who can pass any message you have for them or they have for you from the other plane. Usually these are words of support. People who have passed on to the other plane of existence wish only to offer solace to those left behind because they want them to know they are all right. That is always what they are trying to communicate. "I am all right. I want you to know that. Hear me. Listen to me. I am fine." And people here *seem not to want to open those letters or take those phone calls*. They often prefer to be left in grief.

195

3

Within The Family

Ting-Lao

Families who have members with AIDS must, first of all, under-stand that it is not a terminal illness. It is often a terminal illness right now, but it is fightable. It is conquerable and this will be done. The first step for families is not to say, "Oh, my son or daughter, brother or sister has AIDS, and they are going to die." Families must stop that because that is just signing them away. It is not good.

The next step is for families to do their own introspection and begin having their own relationship with themselves, to find their strength, to find their love for themselves which will give them the courage to go through this illness with their family member.

Illness is a time of change. Each family member can look into themselves to find what they need to change personally in order to relate better with this person. That is the question. Not what they need to change in their personality or in their job or in other aspects of their lives, but what they need to change in their conscious being, in their awareness, in relationship to this family member who has AIDS. This is the opening, the key, the lesson. And then other things in the subculture, such as homeopathy, energy healing, prayer, working with Spirit energies, working with Earth energies, psycho-therapy.

There are many ways to work on this illness. Oftentimes, people will only use one of these methods. The answer, however, does not lie with only one method. Since the entityness of AIDS is very complex, the answer is also very complex. All the avenues must be explored. Families need to provide the energy, the effort, and the work in order to seek out and research these many methods by taking their family member to different therapies and healings, and by being supportive of the person in that way. Do not say, "Oh dear, they are going to die," but rather work in an effort to stop it.

The last step is dealing with sadness and grief, if it is for them to go. If they choose to die from AIDS, then that is what is going to happen. Again, this is where a true understanding of death is important.

4

Taking Responsibility

Ting-Lao

We want to address the responsibilities of those who can infect other people with this virus and we do not want to mince words here. It is an infectious disease, it is an epidemic, and it is of disastrous proportions. We want to ask those people who feel they may have a chance of having been exposed to the virus to get the test. Of course, this does not mean that they will come down with the disease, but they can begin to be more responsible about spreading the disease.

Here we have to be very matter-of-fact because responsibility or irresponsibility can often be a factor in the personality profile of those affected with the AIDS virus. Just as there is a cancer personality or a hypertensive personality, it also appears that there is an AIDS-prone personality, if we want to generalize. Sometimes, irresponsibility is seen in these people. For example, a prostitute who knows that she has AIDS and yet continues to have sexual relations with many men each day so that she can support her drug habit is absolutely and blatantly irresponsible.

We would like to appeal to those people to change and be more responsible. However, because it is so much a part of their personality profile, so ingrained in them, we must ask that people in the society around them please take a step, take a risk, take a chance and talk to them about responsibility. Present the facts to them, inform them that they can carry the disease even though they do not manifest or have symptoms of it.

We must, again, educate people in this way. We must educate people about the facts of having sex in such a way that other people do not get the disease. We must educate them about preventing the giving of it. It is important for what you call the "support-system" people, or people around the periphery of another who is suspected of having AIDS or of having been exposed to AIDS, to take responsibility here, for the society, and for the sake of the future generations.

Soli

Within the homosexual subculture, there is a tremendous emphasis on the mechanics, or the *seeming* mechanics, of how this disease is supposedly transmitted. It has been said by so many teachers that the sexual aspect of this disease and the illness are both symptoms of the underlying disease. We do not see that one is caused by the other, as the disease is not always caused or spread by sex. It is caused and spread by the beliefs, by the self-judgments, the guilt, etc., in the mind while the sexual act is being carried out.

When the individuals focus on what you call "safe sex," it is fine for the time being because it causes individuals to see themselves as being responsible, even if they are focused on the mechanics of the disease's transmission, instead of the underlying cause of the disease that is creating the *need* for that transmission. The mere fact that there is so much focus on the mechanics of how this disease is transmitted means that people are becoming more responsible to self, to partners, to loved ones. It is moving energy into self-responsibility, causing individuals to stop and take a look at their lives and at the repetitive patterns of life that they have been dealing with. And it will move beyond that.

Since the medical model, the mechanical model of how illnesses are spread is so strong within your society, it has become a part of the collective unconscious. So it is only natural that people are moving away from those things which are creating the illness and centering on the mechanical area. However, the movement of AIDS awareness may start from there, but it will eventually spread, as greater understanding moves individuals beyond the apparent mechanics of the disease and into the underlying creation of it, which is within the psyche.

5

Relationships With Others

Ting-Lao

It is important not to expose a person to different strains of the virus. Each virus is mutating into different strains, so one person may have one strain and another person may have another. And two people may feel that it is all right to have a physical relationship since they both have the virus. However, this is incorrect because if each has a different strain it creates double-trouble. It is very important to know that it is not all right to have physical relationships just because you *already* have the virus. You may also contract another strain of virus.

On the physical level, it is difficult to have sexual relationships. One must be responsible and honorable and always tell the person who is interested in having a physical relationship with you that the virus is present in your body. You must do this because the virus *is* contagious. You simply must accept that fact. There are many physical ways of relating that are not contagious.

This virus is more vicious than is talked about. It is getting more vicious, getting more and more energy behind it because of all the fear that is feeding it in the culture, in the world. It is blossoming, just like rodents or insects multiply. The power of the virus is multiplying exponentially just as it is physically spreading exponentially. Physically, one must be more cautious. For example, they talk about safe kissing, safe sex, all these kinds of things. Most of them are too liberal because there is no such thing as safeness when there is this virus. It is simply contagious physically.

So, relationships need to be non-sexual for a time. Touching and stroking the body are very important because this stimulates the auto-immune system, the hormonal system, and the function of the liver. It is very important physically, as well as emotionally.

Laughter is a very important way of moving into relating emotionally. It is difficult to laugh when one has a devastating illness. Laughter causes a chemical reaction in the body that is healing. It is also enjoyable and it is a way to have a relationship when one cannot have the sexual relationship. Just be silly and foolish and laugh, tickle, joke and stroke. Accept the fact that you cannot have any sexual relationships until you move through the disease.

With regard to mental relationships, it is important to relate with people who are in similar situations. We are addressing the gay community here. It is particularly important to talk about this on the outward level, to relate mentally by talking about it while accepting it as something that exists and as something that we can go through, something we can *help each other through.* By not talking about it, by suppression, you use up much of your energy that could be used to fight it. Do not suppress discussing it with someone. There is much too much fear involved here and that is the underlying problem with the whole disease.

Spiritually is also an important way of relating. Many times we advise people to take the time out from having a personal, physical loving relationship and work on friendships, work on one's relationship with oneself and with one's path and with one's God or Goddess.

Acceptance

Dr. Peebles

My friends, often the long-term illness is little more than the opportunity for those around the patient, the families, friends, loved ones, to say, "I love them no matter what they are," not, "I would love them more if they didn't have this illness." Certainly, help them find opportunities to heal. But while that which is your belief might not work for them, it is for you to *hear your reaction* to their illness.

So often you worry so much. Often you say, "Oh, there must be a healing, there must be a way, there must be a way." What you may be doing is guaranteeing that their illness will go on much longer because often they are giving *you* the opportunity to learn to live objectively.

When someone is ill, certainly you make information available to them. But you don't drag them from place to place and say, "Look for a healing here, look for a healing there. Try this, try that, try the other." In that way you are only trying to force a healing upon them so you won't have to face your own reaction to it.

Zoosh

If people were secure within themselves as to who they were, then it would not be necessary to be afraid of homosexuals or gay people. It would not be necessary for them to be afraid and to label these people as "bad" or "strange." It would be possible to say, "Oh, all right, that is who they are. But that doesn't mean that I have to be afraid that I will somehow be affected, or that my loved ones will be snatched from me."

Understand that these people are not pirates. They are not sailing the seven seas in order to convert people with the sword. It is they who *chose* to be who they are. The world sees it as a rebellious nature only because the world does not accept their behavior or who they are. It would be nice for homosexuals if they did not have to hide their love. It would be nice for all of you heterosexuals if you did not hide your love either.

It is a time for loving and accepting each other for who you all are. You as heterosexuals do not have to go out and prove that you are the acceptors of love by trying out the homosexual experience, nor do you have to feel that it will somehow affect you. You are safe. You are secure in who you are. *Let them be that way as well.*

Compassion

Enid

Although AIDS has created a much higher consciousness and a lot more compassion towards the homosexual family, there's also some hardening of the hearts and cries of "wrong-making" from those people who feel that this is a form of punishment from God because homosexuals are not having sex the way it should be done. This attitude shifts off into other segments and it may become worse before it is finished. This lesson of compassion has to be learned across the board, so to speak.

When I speak of compassion, I do not mean to feel sorry for people, as there is no action in pity. It means being able to *identify* with someone's pain and anguish and taking action, helping. In that way, you are also gaining the rewards of that experience without actually having to get the disease. You must remember that you cannot get AIDS unless you have *chosen to have it.*

It's the same thing when you leave your body and you go back and look at your friends in your home Universe. You realize that they experienced everything that you experienced. Your life experience will be shared with every being in existence. Isn't that wonderful? And you are a part of that. No two beings come to experience the same thing; they don't have to, because someone has already done it. So, in a sense, you all are emissaries, sharing experiences and rewards back and forth with your beloved brothers, sisters, and friends in your home Universe.

People are coming together in a very interesting way because of AIDS. We're seeing those attitudes of prejudice and hatred among the doctors and nurses being overcome and dealt with. They're beginning to say, "Well, these people are ill. How can I hate them?" Doctors, nurses, and people in general are having to deal with beings that they really prefer *not to deal with.* And the doctors and nurses are having to see them in a new way, through compassion and love, instead of prejudice and hatred. They see the courage of these people. They see all that courage and all these wonderful things that happen

204

within these people. And their attitudes are changing.

Some patients maintain a sense of anger throughout their illness, but others come into a beautiful place of serenity and are allowing life to happen to them as never before. It is a wonderful experience for some, a very delicious experience for some.

Planting Seeds And Praying For Rain

Master Adalfo

People need to understand that if you can create a little disaster, you ought to be able to create a joy alongside of it. You ought to be able to make it easier. This does not always seem to be that way. Many people still believe in, "no pain, no gain," and this is one of the reasons why they are *still* on the Earth plane. No one ever said life would be easy, that is true. But there is nothing that says life cannot be joyful. Life is joyful and when you see the joy in everything, you no longer need to be here.

I would encourage helping those who are ill to see the Universe as benevolent. Encourage people to open up their inner sight to see what is around them. Give toys, any kind of toys. In your culture (everywhere in the world, really) little toys are gifts of benevolence. Help them to bring out that little child within—not the rebellious one, but the one that just likes to play. *That* little child needs to be encouraged. Read them silly little poems. They are gifts that illustrate the benevolence of the Universe. And, just to give of your time, that is a gift also.

If you have a friend with AIDS who is not knowing about this "channeling" business, you might give them this book filled (as they might see it) with nonsense. Your friend can accept it as a gift of silliness, like a silly little poem. He can read it and laugh if he reads something that he thinks is ridiculous. But what is going to happen as he reads is that certain little ideas are going to begin to plant a seed. Even if your friend throws the book away, or gives it away, saying, "Oh, look at this silly stuff," a seed will have been planted. This will begin to grow very slowly. And he will begin to think about

205

it, not even perhaps consciously. There will be new thoughts on some of the things that have been brought up in this book.

He may be very ill, lying in bed, and may begin to ponder the ideas of lack and abundance. He might just start to think of the good things in his life that he has had and is still having. He might consider, for example, he is in a bed with clean sheets. This is one way of looking at a hospital bed. "I'm in a bed with clean sheets and many people are taking care of me." Or, he can choose to look at the lack in the Universe and say, "Oh, woe is me. I am in bed, sick. No one cares about me." It is exactly the same circumstance. What is different is how he chooses to see it.

All I ask of anyone reading this is that they have enough fertile ground somewhere in which a seed may be planted. And then we pray for rain.

6

Teach The Children Well

Ting-Lao

It is very important to pay attention to this issue of sexuality. Many people become pregnant out of carelessness, unconsciousness, uneducatedness, and unpreparedness. It happens much in the same way as with a venereal disease such as AIDS. You say that it won't happen to you? That is unpreparedness.

For instance, you really feel that you need to have this physical bonding right at this moment, and you are in so much of a hurry that you don't use a safe method, such as a contraceptive or condom. Some strains of the virus can be communicated with kissing. This reality makes it very difficult, not only for teenagers, but also for young adults in their twenties. Again, education is the point here for teenagers. They must live with contraceptives. Otherwise they are in jeopardy of changing their lives in a dramatic way. AIDS is more dramatic than getting pregnant, but it shares the same general truth: one must be prepared.

Maturity is going to come to the young people faster these days because they are going to have to talk to the person that they are interested in having sexual relationships with, and not just fall into bed together. They are going to have to talk and say, "I am concerned about venereal disease, AIDS in particular. Have you had any kind of experience with any person who might have been exposed?" Ask these questions, it must be done. You must be practical. Also, follow your intuitive feeling. For example, one's spiritual guidance will be giving them a feeling of danger or of alrightness. Of course, this is difficult to understand because there are many emotions and hormones involved here that may hinder your receiving the flow of intuition, but we think that it is important to mention intuition. Try to contact your intuitive self or your guides because they do protect and guide you.

It is wise to talk and to use prophylactics and to not just bed-hop. These new behaviors and attitudes are going to change the culture in a positive way. Being promiscuous was on the way out anyway after the sexual searching of the sixties, when venereal diseases spread considerably.

Soli

You have a very Puritan streak in the belief systems of your society of what life is *supposed* to be all about. But, of course, each and every one of you, choosing to be a part of this society, knew that you would be a part of this collective unconscious, knew that you would have to deal with this belief system, this moral structure. It was part of your free will and choice in choosing to incarnate in this time and place. And so it is part of the lesson of experience that you are here to deal with. There is a movement, and we totally support it, to greater freedom of understanding. As we have said so many times, the new society will be based on the three Universal laws, (Allowance, Communication and Self-Responsibility) the second of which is *Increased Communication with Respect.* Increased communication always leads to greater understanding.

You keep your young people in the dark and talk about sex as though it is some black-magic subject that is so dangerous it must not be touched. How ridiculous! Then individuals develop within them these overpowering biological forces and psychological forces because of the secrecy that is being created around sex. Secrecy creates its own energy. If you put the lid on something, the pressure builds up until it blows off. If you put the lid on your children, the pressure is going to build up until they have to experiment and play, and if you

208

do not give them the understanding, then they are going to be playing in the dark. It will be approached as black magic: it will be seemingly dangerous. Therefore, we are totally for increased education, information, and understanding of what the urge is, and how to use it—to understand that *sex does not create disease.*

7

Praying

Ting-Lao

To all the consciousness seekers and metaphysical people, I offer encouragement to you to pray to the energy of healing, so that it will grow and conquer the energyness of AIDS. It will come in a form, such as an anti-viral drug or as some kind of vaccination, immunization or something like this. There will be a big breakthrough, and it has to do with the necessary changes in the consciousness of the people that will, in turn, give more energy to the energyness, the entityness of healing. This must be dealt with on many levels, and with the whole energyness of this plague, so that it does not just repeat itself later on.

Again, awareness of how people limit themselves is one of the shifts in consciousness that must come within the people. There are possibilities of many changes in this life that exist, but because people are so limited and narrow-minded, they cannot accept these possibilities as their reality. They use the same rules of life to live by that the masses have programmed them to live by, which are simply limiting. Open-mindedness is a great key to solving many riddles of life and opens up alternate, qualitative means of living that life.

These are just some of the ways to increase one's awareness that must be acknowledged by the people in order to elevate themselves. There is energy now in the Universe to facilitate this. It is a good time for those who are energy wise in this Age of Aquarius.

What we want to point out is that the work can be done on the energy level. In other words, many times when we talk-talk-talk to people, they are hearing with their ears, but it is going in one ear and out the other. We want to point out here that it is very possible to do work on an energy level in situations like this where another person is not progressing to greater happiness or health. The caring person (in other words, we on the other side of the situation) who sees someone who should be employing certain healing methods on their own, but isn't, can use the energy level through prayer.

We pray to the person's Highest Self each night to please awaken, to please align itself in harmony with the rest of the body. We send much loving and strong energy, sending the energy telepathically and with care. This is one way to help someone when we cannot get through to them on one level. Go ahead and get through to them on the other level. As you go to sleep at night, you can contemplate or think about them so that you can work with them in the energy world of sleep when you are not in your body.

Enid

You can send decisions to others. You can picture others thinking to themselves that they are well and happy. And if it's a good idea to them, they will start following your good thoughts and start thinking like that themselves. So, just go right ahead if you feel that someone needs a little encouragement to think well of himself or to think himself well. You just send it right along. He'll sign for it and then keep it, *special delivery.*

8

Surrendering

Ting-Lao

Oftentimes a person is putting out energy through wanting, praying, and affirming for some growth or passage, and then forgets to surrender. When you are putting out and putting out, it leaves no space for flow to come in. So, I want to remind people to surrender. Say, "This is what I need, dear Universe. This is what I need and I thank you for it and know that it will come in its own just time and space." The Universe does not need reminding. Sometimes a person will proceed with affirmations as it is useful to remind one's own self and subconscious. This is, of course, the main purpose of affirmation, to remind a person that he or she is a worthy and deserving individual.

Sometimes, after people have gone through many processes in order to recreate their own reality, nothing happens. In other words, they are still in physical pain, still lonely, or still experiencing emotional pain. Perhaps things, basically, are not as they want. They are getting older and older, and they tend to become more disillusioned, disappointed, bitter, and angry with God. So, how can they constructively use that energy which is beginning to change?

Many times a person must judge when to surrender and when to take action; that is a great lesson of life. Surrendering still is a necessary part. Many times (especially in this culture) people want to do everything themselves. We have independent people here in

America. We formed our own nation and want to *do it ourselves.* We are very hard-working and intellectual. Many times we feel that we have prevented the flow of God by not trying hard enough or believing hard enough or by doing the "wrong" things.

Part of the benevolence of the Universe is to let yourself accept yourself *as you are,* and say, "I have done my best, and I have done what I feel is just and right, and I accept myself where I am and who I am, for that is perfect." Surrender from that point, and if you are getting disillusioned or disappointed, know that it is all right because that is how it is; for you that is the perfect way. Remember, you are *always* on the path because that is your path.

VIII

Dying

"There is no such thing as death in terms of finality. The real you is energy and Spirit, not form. Even form does not die, but merely transforms itself into something new. . . . Birth and death in the physical realm are basically the same process. At birth you enter from a higher dimension and at death you enter into a higher dimension. You think of death as an exiting, but the only exiting which occurs is when the Spirit exits the physical vehicle. Both birth and death are proceses of entering."

1

Understanding The Process

Kyros

Many people on your planet fear the exiting process which you term "death." In fact, many humans, once they become aware that this process exists, begin to fear. Usually, this begins in childhood when a pet or relative *dies*. Adults try to comfort the child by saying, "Tabby or Fido went to heaven," or "Grandma Pearl went to live with God." But because adults oftentimes mourn so and beat themselves up with guilt by saying such things as, "Oh, I wish I had been kinder to Grandma Pearl," or "I wish I had never kicked Fido or left Tabby out in the rain," children receive this as a statement of finality or that maybe *heaven* or *going to live with God* is not really such a positive thing.

Very small children, because they have recently entered from another dimension and still have some dim recollection of it, have less trouble with the process of death. As a child becomes more programmed by the outer adult world, this recollection becomes locked within his subconscious mind and he begins to perceive as the adults in his world do.

The problem of fear exists because, as children, most adults were programmed by other adults. They see death as something inevitable, something mysterious, something unknown, something filled with pain, and oftentimes as *something final*. And many go through their lives with this hidden fear inside them. You cannot fully live and experience your physical journey if you fear death.

Many people who fear death do so because they do not understand at a deep level that they are *Spirit, not form.* Your form (or body) is only a vehicle to carry you through your third dimensional journey. It is like a spacesuit or life-support system for physical life. If you went to the moon, you'd have to wear a protective suit in order to do your work on the moon. When you returned to Earth or entered a simulated Earth atmosphere, you'd take it off because you'd no longer have need of it. So it is with birth and death. You put on a form when you enter at birth and remove it when you leave at death. It's very important to understand that your vehicle is not you. *You are energy which cannot die or be destroyed, but only transformed into a different kind of energy.* You are Spirit and Spirit contains individual mind with all its levels of consciousness. This is eternal. You were created out of the God essence and God does not die.

Birth and death in the physical realm are basically the same process. At birth you enter *from* a higher dimension, and at death you enter *into* a higher dimension. You think of death as an exiting, but the only exiting which occurs is when the Spirit exits the physical vehicle. Both birth and death are *processes* of entering.

Many do not fear the actual process of death as much as they fear *how* they will die, or *when* they will die, or the physical pain which sometimes occurs prior to the transcendent experience. Oftentimes, how you will die has been determined by your Spirit prior to entering for your own learning, or to teach others or for some karmic balancing. There are no accidents in spite of what you may believe. At higher levels everything has a purpose and a reason and is designed for growth and unfoldment. When an entity dies has to do with his mission. No one ever leaves his vehicle until his individual mission is completed.

I do not wish to sound insensitive about the fears human entities have concerning the process of death. I do understand your confusions and concerns. On the higher dimensions, we do not use the term death. We see what you term as death as merely a *transition* from one dimension to another, from one level of awareness to another. You chose to enter your dimension to learn and to teach so that you might

218

grow and unfold. When this is completed, you move on. Your great Teacher, the Christ, told you about *many mansions* and showed you that death is an illusion through His resurrection. If only you would believe.

As for the pain and suffering that sometimes precede the moment of transcending, these are the illusions your mass consciousness have created. You have created pain and disease and brought them into manifestation, and it has become part of the mass belief system which continues with each generation. You chose to create a world of duality for your growth and unfoldment.

All negative illusions which you perceive are based in fear. The Master Christ was always saying, "Fear not!" Why? Because He knew fear would bind and imprison you and prevent you from experiencing a full and abundant life. He also knew that fear of anything is ego-based, and the ego's main function (as you know) is to maintain and protect the physical vehicle. The ego knows that once the Spirit is released from the vehicle, it no longer has either purpose or power.

I would (if I were able) convince you that there is nothing to fear in the process of transcending. You will be released from fear when you come to the true awareness that the *real* you is *energy* and *Spirit,* not form. You will be released from fear when you reach the awareness that there is no such thing as death in terms of finality. Even form does not die, but merely transforms itself into something new. Ashes and dust return to the Earth Mother and give birth to new life. Nothing dies. All is but transformed. You will be released from fear when you acknowledge who you really are, a Spirit of God, the God Essence. The physical walk is but a short journey in terms of time. There is so much beauty ahead. Fear is released when you align for your own highest good and growth. Fear is released when you replace it with love which is the healing and transforming energy of the Cosmos. This is what your whole purpose is on the Full Circle Journey: *to love, to learn it, to teach it, to be it.*

I would also like to add that sometimes humans fear death because of their attachments to the physical. It is human not to want to leave those people and things which you love and have found joy and pleasure in. Fear will leave if you will remember that those

219

people you've loved and journeyed with are also spiritual beings traveling in physical vehicles and that when you move to another dimension, your Spirits are even more connected and attuned to one another. You don't really leave them. As for attachments to physical things, they will no longer have meaning in a higher dimension. Physical illusions belong to the physical realm. Part of the learning on the physical plane should be to move toward release from attachments to illusions, to the alignment to spiritual reality. Once you have made this transition, there should be no fear. Joy does not cease at the point of transcending, but increases beyond human comprehension.

So, if you fear death, I would say to begin working on your release from fear. Think of yourself as a caterpillar in a cocoon preparing to take flight as a beautiful butterfly into a world of sunshine, or as a rosebud preparing to open into bloom. Though you may not (because of current belief systems) think of it as such, it is a *beautiful* and *joyful* experience and not one to fear.

Soli

The Higher Self has planned out experiences before you came here. You have agreed to have karma with certain individuals that you were going to incarnate with. You have a plan of action, as it were, a schedule mapped out. But when you come here within the physical body, you find that you have this subconscious mind and its beliefs. You have total *free will* and *choice* that allows you to choose to do anything at all. And so, you find yourself moving away from the path that the Higher Self wanted, the path of highest evolution, of greatest growth, of experience–the true path you wanted to have.

If you are too far off course and there is no further way in which the Higher Self can get you back on course, the Higher Self will say, "All right, there is absolutely no point in continuing this lifetime, there is no point in continuing this journey. We're never going to get to San Francisco this way. We're in New York; how can we get to San Francisco? We'll terminate this journey right here." And, so, you decide to leave the Earth plane and you decide that you'll come back and have another lifetime and try again.

Since you are infinite and immortal, you have an infinity of time to do whatever you want to do. If you don't achieve what you set out to do in this lifetime, you will do it in the next life, or in the next, or however long it takes you to do it.

There is no death, my friends. The subconscious mind loves to hang on to the thought that this is all that there is, that once the body goes, it's all over. And even if their lives were terribly miserable, people cling to life desperately until the very last minutes. They cling to it because of their fear of the unknown, their fear that death is far worse than the that which is known.

Death is a matter of rejoicing! How ridiculous are your somber funerals. You should be partying, having fun, and sending the entity on his way with joy instead of with sorrow. When you leave this plane, you are returning to your Spirit brothers and sisters in great delight. They are, in a sense, partying with you. It is fear and the feeling of loss that you will never see that person again, that creates the somber atmosphere at funerals. It is what *you* are feeling, it is what has happened to *you* that creates the sorrow, not what has happened to the person who died. You are really crying for yourselves.

Party, my friends, and rejoice that another has returned home for a time, for a bit of rest and relaxation, before coming back into the *game* again.

When you leave this Earth plane, God does not stand outside of you looking at the life you have led and then punish you by sending you back. Karma does not work that way. Absolutely not! You, yourself, choose your own lives, one after the other. You judge your own selves, and the lives that you have led and you decide to return and balance the energies in some other way. But no one forces you to, my friends. Everything you do upon the Earth plane is free will and choice, totally. You have the choice of how and when to come here. You come as either male or female. You come with parents who either stay lovingly together or who separate and leave you.

Master Adalfo

To help people and their loved ones understand the transition of death, it is not a good idea to talk to them *right away* after the person has died. They cannot hear you when they are in the process of grief. So you talk to someone *before* their family member is going to die. When you know someone is ready to pass, you can talk to the family about the fact that this being has a soul which has taken a trip. This lifetime was that trip. Now he is ready to get back on the boat for his return home. And he will take another voyage here. We *all* have taken many voyages here, and we go back home to review our last trip to make changes for the next one.

You can say that it is as if he stayed in one hotel this time. Next time, he'll try a different one. Let them know this soul has made choices, and that is is important to think about those choices and to communicate with the person about the joys they have shared together. Talk with the person who is dying, if they are able to talk. Let them express their fears and interact with their family. This is not the time to deliver a long lecture about what reincarnation is.

And at the funeral, you can talk about life as a voyage here and how the person is returning home for a rest. You can always give comfort in the sense that you know the person is available to relatives, for a short time, if they choose to communicate. And you can let them know that he or she is *watching* the funeral. To give them hope, let them know what the soul is experiencing on the other side.

222

2

Making Preparation

Dr. Peebles

To prepare yourselves for the transition, be in the light. Live in the light. You are all familiar, hopefully, with the term "hospice." The hospice concept is a rekindling of a concept of creating an environment that acknowledges when our physical life is almost complete. It is a place where you attract light, and where all around you live in light, acknowledging the pain, acknowledging the anxieties, the fears, but calling upon the Guides, calling upon the Higher Self.

If you cannot go to a hospice to die, you should continue living at home and being at your job, telling everyone, "We know I am about to make the transition. I am frightened." Or, you must say, "I'm not frightened, and if you are, go for a ride for the next ten years because I will not have anything except joy and light around me, no matter how miserable and hard this is."

Once you make the transition, if you have not been studying soul communication, of if your intellect has been over stimulated, you will possibly go into a state of sleep. If your religious beliefs are such that you would go to sleep until Gabriel blows his horn, then when you leave the body your soul (or Spirit) will sleep. Oh, it will wake up and look around and say, "Oh, I don't hear a trumpet; I'd better go back to sleep," and it will. But eventually it will get terribly bored waiting for that dumb trumpet and then it will wake up.

And it is your choice. Do you want to sleep when you go to the

Spirit side? Then develop the intellect. If you want to go pure and straight through, study after your soul, study after the *real you*. Give up your old ways, give up your prejudices and your fears, give up your anxiety, and allow everyone else the same privilege. When you leave your body behind, you'll be instantly awake, alert and aware, with no period of adjustment necessary. So, you want to be ready when you pass from this body? Start loving yourself, love everyone and everything and be free.

Ting-Lao

Some people *do not need* to die from AIDS. So many more people die from AIDS than is necessary on the spiritual level. Because of the fear that feeds it, it is like being carried down a roaring river. Once the person joins this group, they are carried away in this river of fear and anxiety and unconsciousness. So, it is good not to join that river in the first place by staying centered and not accepting death. But, if one does get carried down the river with those who are going to pass on out of this lifetime through this illness, then the next step is to deal with the sadness and grief.

The traditional ways are good. The ways that hospices deal with it and through loving communication are both good ways of dealing with it. But the way that most people forget about is through prayer and the connection with God. As you know, there is anger at God. It is one of the stages of dealing with death. One asks, "Why is this (or any disease) happening to this good person?" It is a great wonder, it is a quandary.

There are many reasons why it happens. There is not just *one* reason. Again, it can be a physical reason, as with any disease. It can be that the virus conquered the body in line with the physical laws of the Universe. It can be emotional. Perhaps there was too much fear, so there was not enough will to conquer the energy of the virus. There are many different reasons for succumbing to this AIDS virus or to any disease. But it is the spiritual aspects of this illness that are awakening the culture to the different lessons of death, life and caring.

224

3

When Illness Is Terminal

Soli

It sometimes happens that when an individual has a strong communication or illness, such as a terminal illness, it can be turned around. Why? Because the Higher Self perceives that the individual is learning something new, has made changes within his or her life, has found a way to affect acceptance of that change, acceptance of an understanding of the communication, and is making great changes within his life. He has, therefore, the possibility of a whole new line of experience, as it were, within this dimension.

Then the Higher Self says, "Well, fine. We will have a lot more different experiences now than those which we intended to have when we came here. We do not need to leave now. We do not need to leave and come back within another lifetime. The communication has been understood. The illness no longer needs to be there." And you have what might appear to be a miraculous cure. What has happened is the individual has taken the responsibility for his or her own disease, has done something about it, turned it around and made the changes necessary in their life and has gone forward, no longer with the need for that communication.

Sometimes the Higher Self specifically chooses a lifetime that will be cut short by a certain illness, for the individual has a karmic need to experience, perhaps, a particular physical imbalance. They may have caused such a physical imbalance for another person in a previous lifetime, or judged those who had that physical imbalance. You may have an individual in one lifetime who constantly judged and made fun of someone with a particular physical disability, and because of that judgment has decided to have a lifetime where he experiences *that* particular disability. And so he has *chosen* a lifetime where he experiences exactly the particular projection of energy. And once he has understood that and worked with it, transcended it, then the Higher Self will decide, "Well, perhaps there is no point in staying here any longer. We can leave now. We've had the experience of that particular kind of disability. We will leave and choose a different lifetime."

Again, you will not stop that from happening. You will not stop the Higher Self deciding to end that life. If you find a physical way of prolonging life, and it can be done through mechanical means, then the Higher Self will create what is known as an "accident," which is simply another way of leaving the Earth plane.

Everything, *everything* is free will and choice. You are never a victim. You are not a victim of disease, you are not a victim of a healer. No one can come along and heal you against your will, against your need. *All healing is self-healing*. Understand that and you understand everything there is to be known about healing. It is one of the simplest subjects to deal with upon the Earth plane once you understand it, once you understand that you *are* God. God is not somebody outside of you, sitting in judgment, casting evil spells upon you because you have sinned, because you have gone against the unwritten law. Absolute rubbish, no such thing! You are God. You are God experiencing the Earth plane, experiencing your own creation each and every minute of the day. Once you understand you are God, that you are everything, that you are already one with all life and with each other, that you are always expressing the God force, the God energy through yourself, the I AM experiencing its own creation, then you have no need for illness or disease.

Master Adalfo

People with critical diseases often are better than others at living

226

in the *now*. It comes with an awareness that they don't have an unlimited length of time here. Of course, this is true for everyone. When they begin to face that and acknowledge it, then each day becomes more important. Each day that is left is more important and they become more able to enjoy the pleasures of that day. That is the ideal. Some people fall into that attitude as a natural bi-product of the disease. For others it is more difficult.

For those heavily into the syndrome of lack, they will only see the terrible things to come and not acknowledge the abundance of the moment. It is important to be doing things with these people, things that will help them to see the abundance. Bring them flowers, bring them toys, play games with them, so that for even a few moments, they acknowledge the abundance of *that* moment. If you do not spend time with that moment, how do you know if you have a diamond or a rhinestone? How do you know what it is if you don't take a moment to look at that moment with your jeweler's loupe? Each one of you could use a jeweler's loupe to truly see the day, all the facets, all the light, all the beauty. In this way, you will also get to see if something is a dud. And, if that is true for you, you could just throw it out and concentrate only on the beauty.

Understanding this often is the gift that you find in children who have any disease in which they are dying. Children get that message faster. They *know* what they're here for. And they're often here to just teach others to enjoy each moment, to savor the time that they have together, instead of thinking of the time they will be apart.

The Role Of Children

Soli

Any child who dies before the age of thirteen is a Spirit who has completed all necessary lifetimes upon the Earth plane. These children chose to return to the Earth plane out of service to the parents who needed the experience of losing a child. Before the age of thirteen, a child is not fully formed and is still part of the parents' aura and vibration. After the age of thirteen, all the teaching has been done. The child is fully formed and becomes an adult.

As a Spirit, you incarnate within the physical body anywhere between the point of conception and two months after the actual physical birth of the body. If no individual Spirit wants that experience with those parents or within that society, and if no Spirit chooses that body, there is nothing to keep it alive and it will expire after the two-month period, approximately. This is known as "infant death syndrome" in your society.

The same with abortions. In many cases, the Spirit chooses to be aborted. For example, if a woman aborted a fetus in a previous lifetime and felt tremendous guilt about it, then she would choose to have the experience (in another lifetime) of being aborted herself, just to balance the energy, just to make sure that she did not create any difficulty by doing that in a previous lifetime. You see, it is the belief again. It is because of the guilt behind it. It is not the fact that she aborted the fetus that requires her to be punished. She chose to be aborted in this lifetime to balance that self-judgment.

This applies to every action upon the Earth plane, my friends. There is nothing wrong with any act. It is the *belief* that accompanies it that creates the difficulties. We say again to you, there are no problems in life. There are only events. The problem lies within your mind and how you view the event.

4

Suicide

Dr. Peebles

The topic of suicide is quite monumentous. I, and many on the Spirit side, have a perspective of suicide that does not conform to religious and sociological patterns. I do not see suicide as wrong, or bad, or evil. Suicide is little more than another experience. When suicide is approached, the soul, the Spirit, is not earthbound. It does not live in darkness. It does not find itself caught in the hells. It grows just as anyone who makes the change called "death." Suicide is little more than another choice, one available to all of you. Many accomplish suicide by a life-style or by an attitude.

If one with AIDS says, "Oh, I can't handle this. I'm going to commit suicide," they can accomplish this in a number of ways. They can do this simply by saying, "Illness, I give myself over to you totally, let's get it over with." Within a few days they will make the change called death. They will still accomplish suicide, as you know the term. Those who must witness the suicide will witness it in a clearer, more loving level. They will see it, they will have their same experience, just on a higher level. That's your job, all of you—to have your experiences on the highest level possible. Now, if the person says, "Well, I'm just going to climb to the top of that building and I'm going to jump and land on as many people as I can," then they are gaining the same experience on a lesser level.

If they go out by themselves into the woods, onto the ocean, and

229

make the change called death, swiftly, cleanly, where no one will find them, no one will see them, they are given the same opportunity. They will grow on the Spirit side whether they shoot themselves or whether they just give themselves over to the swift manifestation of the illness. Their experience was to make the change called death at that age, at that time. In short, suicide is not wrong *until* it becomes an escape clause.

The creating of AIDS, cancer, accident, illness, or anything is another escape clause. The majority of illnesses are just another form of suicide. Your society has just not faced it and seen it as a truth. The majority of deaths by accident are usually suicide, and society, through escapism, chooses to call it accident, chance, coincidence.

Tell those with the illness called AIDS to compare their AIDS to diabetes, cancer, arthritis, anything—it is only an illness. It is only an attempt to get out of this life. It is only another *chosen* experience. And if they cannot face it, suicide is acceptable as long as it is done with as much dignity as when they took on the illness.

Soli

Many who commit suicide do so out of the mistaken belief that death is the end of everything. For it is prevalent within your society to believe that this is your one and only lifetime within physical form, and that when you die that is the end of it; then you have lost consciousness forever as it were. That is a *fond hope* of many.

It is most important to realize that there is no judgment against suicide from the spiritual perspective. There is no God judging it to be morally wrong. It is not the worst crime imaginable. It is simply one of the experiences it is possible to have. And it is only the self-judgment, the anger, the resentment, the emotions that are carried through that create difficulty for the individual who has committed suicide. Those that are conscious when they take that action are more able to meet with their guides and teachers, more able to be guided into the higher dimension, more easily able to understand who and what they are, where they are, and so they can move on quite readily. It is not the act of committing suicide per se, that creates any

230

difficulty for individuals. It is the state of consciousness and understanding as that takes place.

But, of course, this applies to what we might call a regular death anyway, or a so-called regular death not by one's own hand specifically. It still depends very much on the consciousness of the individual as to how it is experienced. There are many who die a regular death, who believe that that is the end too, and are very surprised to find themselves waking up. There are many who die in consciousness and have a very easy transition. So, we would say, whether an individual chooses to take his or her own life or not is not *that important.* What is important is the state of consciousness, the understanding.

If the thoughts or ideas of reincarnation are within the subconscious mind, this usually is strong enough to open such individuals to the possibility that they may be in the astral dimensions. Once that thought comes forward, they can then look for their guides and teachers who will assist them from that point on.

On the question of suicide, you must understand that *all,* in a certain sense, are committing suicide. When you watch someone ingesting substances within their life, it is a little easier to see how they are, quite consciously in a certain sense, committing suicide. For the ingestion of substances, drugs etc., any addiction is a slow form of suicide. It is a way of not wanting to have to deal with the experiences of life that you have come here to deal with. It is a way of escape and is perfectly reasonable and acceptable. It is part of the experiences to be had on the Earth dimension. Suicide is only a slightly more obvious form of escape, more catastrophic in the sense of happening more quickly than the slower forms.

Illness itself is a form of suicide. A terminal illness is a form of suicide, for ultimately you are always responsible for your own health and your own life. And if your own health and your own life deteriorates, that is your responsibility, nobody else's. It is impossible to be a victim, so in a real sense, all life ends in suicide. If you see it in that way, then suicide can be seen to be much less a drastic act than you otherwise might see it, not to be morally condemned, not to be judged.

It is for the individuals left behind to bless and release the individual. Do everything in your power, once the individual has left, to speak to them within the spirit dimension, have them begin to understand, even once they have left the physical body, that there is white light around them, there are guides and teachers. Tell them that they do not have to stay around the Earth. Now, if they have been troubled on making their transition, they will be around close to you, they will hear you. And you can do a great deal in assisting them within that process to move on to their next experience.

Now, if an individual terminates their life before they have had the experiences that they came here to have, then it is very likely that they will choose to return to have experiences again, but it need not be exactly the same. The experience of having such an illness is so very much an experience for everybody *around* the individual as much as the individual themselves; in many cases, a lot more so, for the individuals who have chosen to have this illness are here in service. They do not have the need for the karmic experience themselves.

It depends on the consciousness of the soul, and the soul experience it needs, as to whether it is necessary to come back and continue, or to recreate that experience. If you would look at the series of events within the course of such an illness, there is a time period. And throughout that time period there are experiences being had. Because a person ends a life slightly earlier than planned doesn't mean there has not been a lot of karmic exchange taking place and being dealt with. And that final act of taking away ones own life does not necessarily mean that all of that karmic experience has to be relived. It is so much an individual experience, so much an individual question for each soul and each current ego that is incarnated, and there is no generalization that applies to all.

If we were to generalize, we would say that yes, if you take your own life prematurely, then there will be a need to return in another lifetime to experience those things that were not experienced. But where there is already a terminal illness, and a lifetime is approaching its end anyway, that is much less so, much less of a judgment on self in that case. And there is certainly no judgment from any other entity anywhere in the Universe. There is no spiritual judgment on this. It is *most important to recognize this*. There is no morality associated with this. God is not sitting there judging individuals who take their own lives. It is always *self-judgment*. It is the thought form, it is the belief that creates the experience for the individual within the astral dimension, and it is those thought forms that will keep them locked within that dimension until they wake up to the fact of where they are and what they are doing and what they have created for themselves. *Karma is a very over-rated thing within your dimension.*

If you are counseling, or working with an individual who speaks to you about their desire to end their life, there is only one answer, and that is the answer to everything. It is *unconditional love*. It is not for the counselor to judge the individual and their choices. If that individual chooses and wants to commit suicide, it is not the counselor's job to *dissuade or persuade*. It is the counselor's job to love totally and unconditionally, without trying to impose their own belief systems and understandings on the individual being counseled. We are talking about a *saint* here because it is extremely difficult to counsel anyone without getting your own personal feelings and belief systems involved. It is almost impossible. But ideally, this is the way it would be. To be with that individual with such unconditional love that whatever they do is perfectly all right with you.

My friends, remember the full meaning of unconditional love. Unconditional love says, "I do not care who you are, what you are, where you are, or what you are doing. What you are doing in your life is absolutely what you need to do and I am here to support you totally in whatever decision you make. I am not here to do it for you, or to persuade you or to agree with you necessarily, but I am here to support you in the decisions that you make." If an individual has made his or her mind up that it is time to leave this dimension (from the ego point of view), you are not going to stop them anyway. If you try to stop them, you are going to create karma for yourself. You may see them end up in greater suffering. What is that going to do to you? Do you want to persuade somebody to not take their life and have greater suffering?

You see, again, it is looking at it from this point of view of moral judgment of the society. Somehow there is a great stigma attached to

233

suicide and therefore anybody who allows it or accepts it in another individual is somehow aiding and abetting a crime. What nonsense to believe that taking one's own life must be a crime within your society. You would much rather lock someone up under lock and key and observation 24-hours a day than let them take their own life. Is that a better alternative? It is a very strange attitude within your society associated with death. It stems from the need to hang onto life to the last instant, believing that this is the one and only life that you have ever had and you are not going to have any others, and that therefore you must hang onto it and you must force everybody else to hang on to theirs. So you find medical practice trying to prolong life against the will of the individual, against the desire of the individual instead of allowing the natural course of events.

You might look at it the other way, that if the illness were allowed to take its natural course, death would have been much sooner anyway. It is the prolongation of life through drugs and artificial means that creates more problems within an individual. And so, you might see that if that attempt at healing from the external, mechanical, point of view had not taken place, then the life would have been terminated already anyway. And so, of course, within the consciousness of an individual, there is the dichotomy, "Should I make use of every medical advancement, should I try to prolong my life, or should I allow natural events to take place and leave when the body has the need to no longer function?"

In terms of self-healing, of allowing self to be healed, there has to be an improvement in the quality of life, otherwise there is no point in staying on to experience more of the same. If the individual's life is not improving, what is the point of prolonging that life? Do you want to keep somebody alive and in pain and suffering? It all comes back to the fact that the counselor must exercise non-judgment: *The Loving Law of Allowance* for all things and all individuals to be in their own time and space, giving unconditional love and not judging the individual for their choices.

One who hasn't been there can never really understand what it is like except perhaps by going back into previous lives and remembering some experiences they have had of similar nature. And then, of course, once you do that, then you have much greater ability to accept everyone else around you unconditionally anyway, for then you begin to understand what life is really all about. We would reiterate, as we have done so many times, that there is no other purpose to life but experiencing it. And experience is what you are here to do. If you want to terminate that experience of current ego, that is no great problem. The Higher Self will create another ego personality in another time and space if it feels the need to continue that experience. Sometimes it is possible to continue that experience and transmute that experience without coming back into the physical dimension.

5

Euthanasia

Dr. Peebles

Should you be invited to assist someone in their suicide, you must say, "Thank you very much for your invitation. It is your choice, do what you must. It is not my choice to participate." It is not the right of the individual to say, "Oh yes, I'm going to help you blow your brains out." It is the right of the individual to say, "I love you and I respect you, and I give you all of my strength objectively to do whatever you must do," reminding them that if they must make that change called death through suicide, that they take on the choice to do it with dignity, not with horror.

There are times though when euthanasia is acceptable. If the patient has come to the point of remaining on life-support systems, it is not improper for a family member, a lover, or a friend, to refuse the life-support systems. When the loved one has come to the point of losing consciousness, losing control, and is no longer there, and the body is kept alive through drugs, if you can see that the being is already on the Spirit side, then *allow* the change called death. Yes, euthanasia is at that point, acceptable. But if the person is still there and just doesn't want to face their problem, euthanasia is not acceptable.

Soli

If you, as an individual, are requested to assist someone in this experience of suicide, it then becomes a matter totally of individual conscience and consciousness. With all the aspects of condemnation of the rest of society, it is like any euthanasia, any *mercy killing* as you so aptly put it. You find individuals who assist in a mercy killing being imprisoned for the rest of their lives for an act of kindness. It is society's attitude. An individual of whom such a request is made has all these aspects to deal with within self in coming to a decision. Ultimately it can only be with the inner being, with the inner feeling. As we have said, there should be no judgment on these things. There should be no judgments on other individuals in any way, shape, or form. But the way your society is right now, there is that tremendous difficulty in assisting an individual in this way.

It is very difficult to answer this question without being an advocate. What we are trying to do here is to answer these difficult questions and keep the balance so the individual sees his or her own way. We do not wish to say, "This is the way it should be." But, we would suggest that you look at it this way, that you do not *actively* take an individual's life. But then, on the other hand, you do not try to prolong it either. And there is a very big difference between *allowing* an individual a natural release from the physical body in comfort and ease than there is to actively seek to terminate that life. And it is very much an individual decision, and there is no way that we can say, "This is the way it must be."

IX

Raising Levels Of Consciousness

"If you hear different things from different teachers, go within yourself and ask which teaching most suits your needs at this time. There is only one teacher, my friends, and that is yourself. . . . We Spirit Guides can only give you a perspective, a different point of view, a different understanding. . . . The only guideline we would give to you is that those beliefs which limit you, get rid of them. Accept those that open up your limitations. . . . Always widen your horizons."

1

Examine Your Beliefs

Soli

Raising your level of consciousness means becoming conscious of that which is presently unconscious. All those belief systems which you have stored within your subconscious mind are brought to the surface and examined honestly.

In the gay community, it means to examine honestly the fact that you do believe what society is telling you, that you are a crime against nature, that you are a sin against God, and that you must be punished for it. That is a deep-set belief. It is so deep down that most of you do not acknowledge it; but it is there. So it is with all the other beliefs about the self, all these thoughts that keep recurring day after day throughout your life.

Our fondest example is, "I cannot afford." Friends, ask yourself, how often in a day do you say to someone, "I cannot afford that, I cannot afford this. I cannot go out to dinner. I cannot afford the time." What are you telling yourself? Daily, day in and day out, you are affirming your limitations. You are affirming that you are a limited individual, that you cannot have what you need to experience and to enjoy yourself. It is an affirmation that you are making constantly and it stems from your parents' beliefs about certain things. You see an individual of a certain racial type and immediately a judgment springs to mind and it goes almost unnoticed.

You are to become conscious of those beliefs. As they occur, ask

241

yourself, "Is this serving me? Do I need this? If the answer is "no," turn it around. Bless and release the thought. "Thank you for giving me what I needed to have up to now." Don't fight your subconscious minds, my friends, you are working *in harmony* with them. Become conscious of those thoughts that are of no use to you anymore. Then bless and release them, turn them around.

For example, the "I cannot afford." If you see some object in the shop window that you desire, you look at it and say, "I cannot afford that," then you will never have if for you are affirming your own limitations. However, if you look at that object and say, "Hmmmm, this object is mine. Obviously I don't need it right at this moment because it is not in my hand. When I truly need it, it is in my hands." It is a totally different vibration. You are not limiting yourself. You are widening your vibrations, allowing the possibility. You see, my friends, the only limitations that you have in life are those which you believe.

There is no such thing as a miracle. Each and every one of you can walk on water. Each and every one of you can transfer yourself to any point on the Earth plane instantly in time or space. Why can't you? Because you believe that you cannot. You believe that it takes a very special individual, or much training, or whatever. It is belief. Let go of those limiting beliefs.

You will be constantly challenged, my friends, time and again. You can listen to another Spirit Teacher who says things very differently from Soli. You will be challenged if you believe everything that Soli is saying and it becomes part of your belief system. Those beliefs will be challenged by someone else. There is no absolute reality, no absolute truth. Ultimately there is only what *you* believe. If you hear different things from different teachers, go within yourself and ask yourself, "Which most suits my project at this time?"

There is only one teacher, ultimately, and that is yourself. There is no one higher than your own Higher Self. No one knows better for you what is right for you than your own Higher Self. We can only give you a perspective, a different point of view, a different understanding. But we do not claim to have the absolute truth. Examine your belief systems. The only guideline we would suggest to you is that those beliefs which limit you, get rid of them. Those that open up your limitations, accept them. Know that they too will fall by the wayside as more and more further widening and expansive beliefs come along.

Zoosh

Remember that God is not afraid. Also remember that each and every one of you are aspects of God. You are children of God in that sense. There is no definite reason to perpetuate a fear of your fellow man. Be a little more friendly and a little more kind to yourself, then friendly and kind to your loved ones and let it spread from there.

Pay attention to what goes on around and about you. Do not assume the attitude that if your brother or sister is in discomfort that it is only their doing. If you will allow the idea to enter your mind that discomfort is natural and normal, then you will open yourself up to experience discomfort and allow others to do so with the absolute certainty that it is normal. Conversely, if you would allow yourself to believe that comfort is normal, you will be more accepting of your own experience of comfort and your own experience of the comfort of others. Allow yourself to believe that comfort is normal, that ease is normal, and that safety is normal. In this way you will literally change your world and allow your world to change around you.

2

Taking Self-Responsibility

Soli

The Age of Aquarius is an age of changing consciousness. It is an age in which there is a greater understanding of many things: that your essential self is your God Self, that everyone is here by choice, and that everyone is entitled to live by their own belief system, since all are equally as valid as your own. You accept another's belief at its face value, whether or not you agree with it. This allows you to communicate more deeply with one another.

Above all, in this age of changing consciousness, the New Age, individuals must take more responsibility for themselves within their lives. That is what the Age of Aquarius is all about: self-responsibility.

In today's society, just the opposite is true. If you stub your big toe on your neighbor's doorstep, you sue him because you blame him for your own error, it is all his fault, not yours. Blame someone else, be a victim. This is a growing tendency in today's society. There are a great many people who feed on this attitude as it hands over more power to them, and they are the ones who are in power and have control. Members of society have handed their power over to others. Not only do they blame others, but they depend on others to decide for them also, to rule. So many people have given over their power of self-responsibility to others with the attitude that they do not know how to live their own lives, that they need someone else to lean on, to organize life for them, to make laws for them, to control them, as they are not capable of doing for themselves. Of course, this allows those who love power to have control in all aspects of life, political, religious, legal and more.

The more individuals who take responsibility for themselves and for their own lives, the more of a backlash is going to arise from those people who are in power, in control now. They are going to feel that their power is being taken away. Much conflict will arise from this, my friends. You will be a part of this conflict to the extent that you perceive or judge that what they are doing is wrong. If you get caught in judgments, then you pull yourself right into the vibrations of those whom you are judging. Allow yourselves to continue doing what you need to do by following your own dictates, and allow others to do the same, and do not judge them. This is how consciousness changes, yours as well as society's.

Those people who take responsibility for themselves will experience a higher vibration, since they are following their need for growth and experience, which is necessary for their evolution. Some people will not take responsibility for themselves because they do not need this experience for their growth at this time. There will be other planes of vibrations that will become the "playground for juvenile delinquents," as one of our friends from the Spirit plane has called it. There will be other opportunities for those people who still require that kind of experience. These individuals have not dealt with their karma of previous existences and still need to go through certain experiences, which may be judged as negative, in order to evolve. This is not wrong or negative. They are not failing to move to a higher energy level because they are not developing fast enough. Everyone is infinite, immortal, eternal, and universal. Time does not exist. So, if you do not do it in this lifetime you will in the next. If you do not do it on the Earth plane, you will do it somewhere else. It will be done. It is as simple as that. There is no judgment upon this. There are so many who look upon the changes of the Earth plane and judge so harshly, and say "Change or otherwise you will suffer." It is not that at all. Suffering, of course, always comes from the subconscious belief systems. No one is going to be punished because he did not reach a certain level. It is simply a matter of choice. You chose not to reach a certain level. You choose to do it in this lifetime or the next, or the next, or the next.

This is the paradox of spiritual growth: nothing is right or wrong. Nothing cannot or should not happen, for you are infinite and have an infinite amount of time in which to do it. Ultimately, it will happen. From a worldly point of view certain things seem so important to you, but seen from a higher perspective, from the spiritual point of view, nothing is more important, nothing is less important.

Working on the self is important, however, as that is a movement towards the spiritual dimension. Self-growth raises the consciousness in others, allowing them to grow also. It also assists the Spirit of the Earth in its process of incarnation. This is why you find so many teachers, such as us, at this time, working within the physical dimension, trying to bring forward different perspectives, trying to persuade more and more individuals to work upon themselves and raise their vibrations, for it will raise the vibrations of all.

3

Understanding
The Collective Awareness

Kyros

You all know that the "Hundredth Monkey" concept is based on the premise that at the onset, a certain number of entities have a particular awareness. At a certain point, if only one more entity is given the awareness, it can cause the awareness to touch almost everyone no matter where they are located. It's a psychic mind-to-mind connection.

The tendency, of course, is to consider that any awareness will always be a positive quantum leap in man's perception. You must remember, however, that awareness is awareness and is neither positive nor negative of itself. It is neutral and it is your perception which labels the new awareness as positive or negative. Once an awareness, no matter what the awareness is, reaches a critical point within mass consciousness, this awareness can touch everyone's individual consciousness. You must also remember that if the awareness is accepted, it can then be brought into manifestation.

With this disease you call AIDS and with cancer and some of your other diseases, the leap in consciousness to the awareness of these diseases has occurred. Not only has the awareness of these diseases reached the critical point in mass consciousness, but they have been *accepted* by mass consciousness. As individual consciousness accepts the awareness perceived by mass consciousness, the individual egos perceive the new awareness through the eyes of fear and ignorance.

Not only have you accepted the new awareness, but you have perceived it negatively.

Mass consciousness is now generating great fear and hysteria, which is causing the physical manifestations of the disease to increase upon your planet. It is a question of fearing that which you do not know or understand. You cannot know and understand until you release yourself from fear. Ignorance is but fear blocking reason and enlightenment.

By comparison, the numbers of those who fear are greater than those who do not fear. This is why the physical manifestations are increasing rapidly. There are a few who do not instill the new awareness with fear, and as they increase in numbers, they will trigger another awareness in mass consciousness and you will call it a "cure."

For example, are you really sure that the Salk and Sabin vaccines practically wiped out the disease called polio? Or did mass consciousness accept a new awareness that the vaccine would work? In other words, was it the vaccine which worked or was it the belief by mass consciousness that caused it to work? It is difficult for me to make you understand not only the power of individual mind, but of collective mind as well. Human entities *manifest* what they give power to. If they render power through fear they will produce negative manifestations.

So much of what I teach is based on the truth that you are responsible for your individual world, and that your individual mind, being part of collective mind, is in part responsible for your total external world. This is why so much emphasis has been placed on learning to think properly and positively and of taking responsibility for the creation of your own individual world rather than looking outside yourself at the externals. Your life is how you create it to be and your world is how mass consciousness creates it to be.

As an individual mind, you do not have to buy into everything which the collective mind promotes. This does not mean that you will not be touched by the various illusions created by collective mind. You will always have a shield of wisdom, knowledge, and enlightenment available if you do not block them by fear.

248

Collective mind tends to be fear-oriented and this is why I have stated before that it is the *individual that evolves,* not the masses. It is an individual monkey who first washes his potatoes to remove the sand from them. Others then release their fear and follow his ways and add their strength of energy to the action until the hundredth monkey is reached and the breakthrough into a new collective awareness is made.

Remember also that the hundredth monkey would have no value were it not for the first fearless monkey willing to separate himself from collective mind and for the second, third, fourth and so on willing to move out and experiment with new thinking.

As for the disease called AIDS, it might be helpful if you would raise your awareness and seek to understand why mass consciousness has created a disease which breaks down the human immune system. Symbolically try to discern what collective mind is saying and why it is bringing this into manifestation on your planet.

Zoosh

At the time of World War I, there was no real consciousness of *one world.* It took a war, a drama, to draw attention to the idea that everyone was living on one world, one planet, and was involved in some massive struggle together. That consciousness, developed those many years ago, was a parallel experience to the current experience of AIDS, even though it was not a disease. War is essentially a man-made disease. It is a way of attacking the bodies of your fellow beings for beliefs that those fellow beings are threatening you. It is very basic, very simple. As long as you believe that your fellow man somehow brings threat to you, you incorporate the belief that you are not safe. It all comes down to that. So, you will create, at various times, demonstrations that safety is something that must be created from within, not simply by controlling your environment.

World War I was a massive attempt to control the environment; the environment being mankind. You can see that it was not a war to end all wars, though it is referred to as that. Instead, it became a war that *began* world wars. The lesson did not sink in. Understand that

249

at moments of extreme consciousness change, you will create demonstrations, just as you have created world wars.

So you have created a worldwide disease in the form of AIDS, which, at its very low key level, did not seem to be threatening but one single segment of your society. The disease will, in time, seem to be a bit more threatening, just before the cure is upon you.

Every few years or so you go through a massive consciousness change. In the early 1900's, the mass consciousness change was that you were of one world, not just separate fragmented countries. People who had never heard of France became aware of France. People who had never heard of other places became aware of them.

Now the objective of the consciousness change is to integrate into your life the spirituality that you experience in church on Sundays, or in temple on Fridays or Saturdays, or as your religious practice throughout the week. In other words, incorporate your Spirit-God self into your day-to-day self.

4

Communicating With Your Higher Self

Working With The Subconscious Mind

Soli

If you would have the highest possible evolution within this lifetime, then you would choose to accept authority and responsibility for your own life. You choose to say, "I will live my life according to the way I need to, what is best for me." Then comes the question, what is best for you? Only your Higher self, *your own* Higher Self can tell you that. And how does it do that? If you do not listen, it tells you by disease. You do not have to have that communication through disease, you can communicate with your Higher Self first. You can do this through meditation, through relaxation, by talking to yourself, talking out loud, talking to your Higher Self, communicating, affirming, visualizing, creating within your life, working with your intuition, following your *feelings,* and not your intellect.

To be a bit more specific, there is really only one thing to do, and that is to *let go and listen.* You see, sometimes you are willfully, quite willfully, not wishing to take notice of that guidance even when you hear it. You hear that guidance, you know very well, you feel strongly that you *should do* something, and you willfully decide you are going to do the opposite. You do not want to take notice of that guidance. You see, my friends, it is the subconscious mind that brings forward the fears and doubts, frustrations, anger, all the emotions, all those things that would stop you moving forward in the direction you are being guided to go.

KEEPING THE STATUS QUO. The subconscious mind is dedicated to the status quo. It would much rather maintain the condition of discomfort that it is familiar with than open up to the possibility of greater discomfort, even though there is a possibility of much less in some changed situation.

The subconscious mind does not like change. Your memory is a storage of all that you have received through your five senses. Whenever a new sensory input is put into that, all the other storage areas are shaken up a little. It is a discomfort within that memory, the subconscious mind. It has to re-assess all those things which are already there, and this is difficult. It is an organ of fixed knowledge with very little fluidity and change. And so anything new within the subconscious mind creates great upheaval.

And so, when your Guides and Teachers come forward with guidance, the subconscious mind does everything it can to blanket that communication. While you are involved in thinking, allowing the thoughts of the subconscious mind to rattle around, the energy of the Higher Self is filtered, it is stopped. It is rather like a filter over a ray of light. The more you can stop that subconscious from being busy, from thinking, the more the energy of the Higher Self can come through. And from that communicating channel (the Higher Self) comes your guidance from your Higher Self and from those that are working with your Higher Self within the Spirit plane—your Guides and Teachers.

There are many techniques for working with the subconscious mind. Here are a few:

(1) WORK WITH DISCIPLINE. It has been said that discipline is the negative, it is the darkness and that the Higher Self and the communication is the positive (the light of many forms). The darkness of the discipline attracts the light of the Higher Self. Therefore, more of the Higher Self can be drawn through from the discipline of relaxation and meditation. Take the same time, the same place for meditation each day, preferably in the morning when you have just awakened into the physical body. You are still somewhat out, not

252

fully back under the control of the subconscious mind. You have come back from your travels in your sleep state.

(2) MEDITATE AT THE SAME TIME, SAME PLACE each day, for that disciplines the subconscious mind, allows it to feel, "Yes, now we're doing the same thing. Yes, I understand that. That's not change, that's the same thing. We did that yesterday and the day before. No difficulty there." And so the subconscious mind is lulled into a false sense of security so the Higher Self can come through much more easily.

We do not wish to imply that the subconscious mind is an enemy. It is not. It is essential. It controls your body, keeps your heart pumping, keeps you breathing, controls the muscles when you walk along the street. And so you learn to work with the subconscious mind, not against it. You simply work with it, understand its power and learn to reprogram it by affirmation, by visualization.

Now, within that meditation (same time, same place), the visualization helps to center the subconscious mind, helps you to keep it busy on some task (such as visualization) that it is familiar with. It does not then come forward with so many ideas and thought forms. The *stronger* you can visualize an object, the less you have thoughts darting around your head.

(3) SPEAK OUT LOUD TO YOUR GUIDES, addressing them by name. This creates a vibration in the subconscious. The subconscious feels that it is talking to an individual upon the Earth plane. It is just as though you were conversing with someone present in the room. Speaking out loud has a similar effect. Also, it slows down your words, slows down your thought processes. Likewise, write down the answers to the questions that you put forward. As you work with the pencil, the muscles work writing laboriously each word. This slows down the thought processes. You are so busy catching each word, writing it, that the mind does not have the time to go flitting off into a thousand and one different directions before it catches the communication. All these things, practice and discipline, allow this communication to grow rapidly.

253

The Search For Reconnectedness

Dong How Li

This planet and all the beings who share it are in such great longing for being whole again, for being reconnected. Each of you is longing for that connection in yourself and reconnectedness with others on the planet. The planet too is aching for this to take place. When you have such great pain, it cries out enormously in silent ways for any kind of theory, any kind of idea that might show an alternative. Even if they resist, people are fascinated by the idea that they are part of a natural cycle, just as nature is. People have seasons, too; only their seasons occur in different bodies. It's their soul which remains the same, going through each of the seasons. People crave this reconnectedness; but only when they have gone through the whole cycle can they attain conscious awareness of the whole, of wholeness. Then they become truly reconnected.

For example, look at the hero who goes on a quest because something at home is not quite right. The answer is elsewhere. So, he goes off and looks and has all kinds of adventures, some of which scare him, and he calls for help. After so many adventures, he feels very confused and doesn't know quite where he is or how to put all those experiences together. Then despair arises and the hero goes into the dark night of the soul, so to say. Something usually fails, the ship falls apart or the crew mutinies and then all the doubts, the questions and the fears come to the surface, all the "demons" are faced.

That is your anguish. That is where this planet is now, in case you hadn't noticed. All the demons that are inside are forced to express themselves outwardly because humanity doesn't want to look inside. People want to fight instead. This is why it is so important for you in the New Age to be willing to look inside. That is what you must change first. In order for the outside to be changed, the inside must be changed. And those of you who do change inside will greatly affect the people around you, and more of them will change. It is like a chain reaction.

When you come out of that "dark night of the soul," you know that

254

all those terrible things that happened out there were reflections of your own self, the parts of you that were out of balance. Your inner state reflects in the world around you. When you bring yourself and your experiences into balance, then you come out of that "dark night." You are able to move faster, more directly and forward on your path. You now know your path is the path that leads you home again, the end of the story.

At that point, you have gone through all your "seasons." You feel whole, unified; you know connectedness. People are looking for that connectedness now, that feeling of wholeness and of unity in their lives. The churches are not giving it, nor is the government, nor are society, economics or advertising. As a matter of fact, they are continuously trying to separate you from yourself, to get you to have your "adventure" down their lane. The world, in general, is a great distraction for those seeking wholeness. Remember that the answer lies within while the world tries to lure you out.

Keeping A Journal

Dr. Peebles

I suggest that you keep a journal every day, a journal of awareness. The journal should include notes of how you feel physically and mentally when you awaken every morning and notes of your dreams and astral projections. You might say, "Well, I do not dream." But you do have body responses, which are stimulated so often by your dreams. Write down those reactions–the dry throat, the pressure behind the eyes, the stiffness in your muscles. I hear some intellectuals saying, "But I always have stiffness in my muscles." That is not the point. Write down the new stiffness; for it is indeed new each day. If you do not embrace that understanding, then the stiffness will never be healed.

Along with the journal of awakening, include your sudden awarenesses during the day. I don't mean for you to carry your journal wherever you go, but do have pieces of paper on hand. At the end of the day, take these pieces of paper and write them into your journal

255

and say, "I remember, this is the note about the cloud I saw while I was stopped at the traffic light. Here's a note of that interesting man I saw washing the windows of the thirty-seventh floor. Many saw him, but did not perceive him." Also, write down the things that you have left undecided each and every day. Write down those things that need attention, for you have made decisions.

Many of you make decisions and have no idea of the responsibilities and directions of your decisions. Write down your decisions and your indecisions. You will find that this process will bring you toward a twenty-four-hour-a-day awareness. One of your greatest roles in this life is to embrace conscious awareness twenty-four-hours a day. You will attain such a state of awareness that you will be able to maintain consciousness during your sleep, during your meditations. You will be able to maintain consciousness and have rest and rejuvenation.

Master Adalfo

A journal is an excellent idea for keeping an account of your feelings every day. Write down your feelings, by all means. Also, a dream diary is a good idea, where you keep track of your dreams. After a while, you will be able to communicate with yourself through your dreams.

Another way is to allow yourself some quiet time every day, five or ten minutes, where you can simply sit quietly and do meditation, prayer, and make communion with Spirit. You can ask your Higher Self questions, and then make the space to hear the answers. If you do this exercise of writing down those questions and writing down the answers to them, you must continue to do this for a long period of time before you *know* where the answers are coming from, so that you are confident that it is, indeed, your Higher Self. You must have perseverance. Do not give up.

Another way of getting in touch with your deeper self is through ceremonies or rituals. Be creative and devise ceremonies for yourselves to begin and end each day with—like lighting a candle, or picking a flower and putting it in a vase. Some people need this in their life because it is a way of putting form on their life and their world. It tells them, "This is a new day. I cannot undo the past and I cannot worry about tomorrow. Today is the day I am dealing with. This is the day I shall live." And when they do that, they get in closer harmony with what is going on with them that day. So, devise little ceremonies, whatever speaks to you. You will have to experiment. Some people seem not willing to do that. They try something once and they say, "Oh well, this isn't working." And of course, they don't give it enough time to know. They decide after two days that it isn't working. They have not very much patience. They may wish to try something else. Don't give up all together trying to communicate with yourself. A little persistence may be in order.

Living In The Here And Now

Dr. Peebles

My friends, you should, each and every day, *bless* the opportunities of living the day as if it is a new lifetime. Bless each day. When it is over and done, bless it as if it were equal to a previous incarnation. Take each and every decision of the new day as if it is new, totally new, even when it is based on something you put into motion yesterday. Remember, every decision that you have to make also exists in the reality of other people, and they have changed just since yesterday. You, also, have altered just since yesterday. No matter what was perfect and right in your experiences yesterday, you must now re-evaluate, and your decision must be based not on what it would have been yesterday, not on what it might become tomorrow, but on what is *best for the moment*. For whatever decision you make now will change by tomorrow. So, if you have your hopes based on what it will evolve into, you are deluding yourself, getting caught in webs and shadows.

If you are to embrace your oversoul totally, make your decisions apply to life in the current moment, the current time, the current space. You will find greater peace tomorrow, greater ability. You will find the objectivity that you all claim you are working toward. And I

257

might say to those reading these words: unconditional love is another term that is so terribly *misunderstood* in this era, and it is worthy of as much research as the concept of creating individual reality.

By living in the moment, you will find a clearer understanding of unconditional love. Unconditional love will only manifest, my friends, when you live in the current moment with your husbands, your wives, your lovers, your co-workers, your projects, your children, your friends and your relatives. Love them not according to what they might be or what they could have been, but love them for what they currently are.

5

Laying Tracks For Yourself

Enid

Think about life as laying tracks in front of you. Just before you step, you put a track out there for yourself to walk on; you continue to keep putting it there. Now once in awhile, during our lives, we say, "It's hard putting out my tracks. I'm tired of planning my life and working on it." So you just sort of take chance–then you take the chance of falling through the cracks. The cracks can be really deep, deep and narrow and you find yourself looking up and you only see a little piece of sky. You don't really see what else is up there.

Laying out tracks helps you to live in the *now*. Being willing to experience at this very moment is living in the now. You can look at now, then, and way out into the future all at the same time. You have great scope as a being. So, if you've laid your tracks and you say, "This is what I want to have: I want this general thing to happen for me and I want somebody out there waiting to be my partner too." You can put that out there too. And you can put it close to you, the sooner you want it to happen. As you walk along the tracks, you don't continue to put those things out the same distance as you walk on your tracks; you're literally bringing them to you. You bring things to you that you want. That makes your power grow more and more and it puts you more in charge of what's happening. So you don't have to put vast great amounts of effort on it.

You can live life from any kind of viewpoint you want to. First of all, the big viewpoint that you want to look at is: how do you want to live your life? Do you want to live your life from the edge and just take chance? There are many people who do that: mountain climbers, race car drivers, hoboes; they never know what's going to be next. They lay great plans for their life. Even the hobo, he lays great plans for jumping onto that train or whatever he's going to do, all the people that he wants to meet at the next stop. There are a lot of plans laid, even for those who want to live in chance. They're living in the now, but they're also living in the future winning that game they're planning. There's nobody that can live totally in what you call the now and have any success or feeling of accomplishment.

I think perhaps the first person who said that was a person who realized that we can't always live deciding to become something, that we are something *now*. And we can love the flowers that are in the room now and the light that's here now and the energies and people now, but also we have attention on, "Tomorrow's going to be a wonderful day and this is what I'm going to do and this is all happening out here." That doesn't mean your full attention isn't going on here, but you're also laying your tracks. It takes so little effort to do it. Just put them there. But if you're always thinking you've got to have this thing that you don't have and you've got to have that thing you don't have, that's part where living in the now is a good idea. To enjoy what you have now, to be *happy and content* with what you have now. Let it serve you good and realize it for the beauty that it is.

Sometimes beings confuse worry with concern about where they should lay their tracks. Worry is not caused by true worry about the future, but about worry over the past. So, if you're talking about worrying, you could put everything you'd ever need out in the future and that wouldn't stop your worrying unless you've handled your past. One good way of handling your past is to take scissors and cut it off. Say to yourself, "That's the end of that!" Just one little snip and your past is gone. Worry in the future is really worry of the present; it's fear of now. The next minute is a tiny future.

Dong How Li

My whole purpose is to try to help people be in the present because I believe that if you're there, and firmly, you'll get to the future with no problem. The problem is *people want to get to the future without being here.* That doesn't work. If you get to the future, what are you going to enjoy? You can't be there either, you will be wanting to be somewhere else.

Welcome Change

Taulmus

Many people fear change and view it as a threat to their security. In truth, change brings the opportunity to know that material security is but a fleeting thing and that the stability which has lasting value is anchored in the divine expression within, which is ever expanding into unlimited freedom, unlimited love.

Change brings a time for re-evaluation of one's life and a chance to hone new skills and develop latent talents and abilities. This you do by tuning into the knowledge of the whole which is as near to you as your breath, your heart beat. To tune in is to still your thoughts, to sense your connection with all life, to listen to the truth of your being. It is then that you will simply know what corner you need to turn in your life, what needs forgiveness, and what needs unloading or leaving behind. In this way, you free up new energy, creative energy that brings to the fore talents you never before knew as your own.

261

X

Hope For
The Future

"You are existing in a very interesting era of the planet Earth. Your vibrations are increasing, speeding up. . . . Even your slightest belief system is going to demand realignment, restructuring, re-evaluation. . . . It is a time to willingly look deep into the recesses of human consciousness. It is a time of taking chances, a time of finding how to integrate your spiritual philosophy, your spiritual code of ethics, with your daily practice of life."

1

Closing Comments

Jesus of the Light

My friends, as witnesses you can do a great deal to spread the word of education and love for those who experience the disease of AIDS. Do this not only for those who witness it, but also for those who observe it, as well as for those who judge it. It is through friendliness and love and appreciation, through acceptance and forgiveness, that this disease and all diseases will be reestablished in harmony in the physical self. This disease will not be conquered. If it is conquered, then it will again be Armageddon. If, on the other hand, it is loved into re-energizing as something else, not going away to be a disease elsewhere, but having its energy re-energized as comfort, harmony, self-love, friendship, joy, and awakening light, then this disease can be a *gift* in disguise. For that which points out a discomfort in you and a discomfort in society as a whole, can truly be a friend in disguise.

Taulmus

Many on your plane of existence are awakening to the realization that the old ways of pain, suffering, agony, and distress no longer work. For those who are remembering the truth of their total being, there is *new* life, *new* hope in a world still mired in conflict and suffering. Pain, my brothers, need not be your lot and you don't need to sacrifice yourselves to disease and ill health.

Dr. Peebles

Dear ones, it is oh-so-important for you to understand that you are existing in a very interesting era of the planet Earth. Your vibrations are increasing, speeding up. You are under tremendous influences of the astrological configurations of the moment. You do not have to be caught in the confusing webs of this moment. If you will embrace your spiritual code of ethics, you will be able to live in the world as you know it, and turn it into security for yourself and others. So, rather than being caught in a confusing era, you will be able to show the way for all to make the best of the changing time.

Now, I do not believe in everything and anything for everyone. You all must reach a level of awareness of who you are physically, mentally, and spiritually. Create an atmosphere within yourself so that you will know intuitively what is best and right for you, that which will keep you growing and expanding toward the greatest light. Do you see? As soon as you find yourselves plateaued and feeling comfortable, you've got to know that you've missed the boat some place.

Life is a delight, enjoy it. Life was chosen by you. When it is the most difficult, know that you are closest to the fulfillments that are rightfully yours. When you are feeling a "little bit crazy," know that you are closest to the Spirit.

Fear not the experiences of life. Fear not yourself. Fear no one or anything, for you are the light and you are the power. There is nothing imagined or in the Spirit that can harm you. Call upon your Higher Self, enjoy the challenges, for they are only that. You have free will, manifest it. Call upon your Spirit Guides and Teachers. Create abundances individually and collectively. Go your way in peace and love and harmony. May the Gods and the kingdoms bless you!

Master Adalfo

Remember that is is not necessary to rely only on yourself to heal yourself, but that does not mean you could not add to the process. As I have said, "Healing is loving and loving is healing." So if you are going to heal yourself, that means you must love yourself. And let there be *much* more of that.

Ting-Lao

This illness has come to give people with AIDS a different space and time in their lives. Their lives have changed. It cannot go on in the same way, with the same kinds of relationships. Relationships must change and the change should be from the emotional, physical, or social level, into the more inward relationship with oneself, one's deities, and with others through friendship. We encourage you all to take some time out and create other kinds of relationships, particularly with one's own Spirit-Self. The bonding of the personality-self with the Spirit-Self is particularly comforting at this time.

Zoosh

Remember that God is not afraid. Each and every one of you are aspects of God. You are children of God in that sense. There is no definite reason to perpetuate a fear of your fellow mankind. Begin by just being a little more friendly to yourself and kind to yourself, and then friendly and kind to your loved ones and let it spread from there.

Pay attention to what goes on around and about you. Do not assume that if your brother or sister is in discomfort, it is only their doing. If you will allow the idea in your mind that discomfort is natural and normal, then you will open yourself up to experience discomfort and allow others to do so in the belief and absolute certainty that it is normal. Understand, if you would allow yourself to believe that comfort is normal, then you will be more accepting of your own experience of comfort and your own experience of the comfort of others. Allow yourself, then, to believe that comfort is normal, that ease is normal, and that safety is normal. In this way you will literally change your world and allow your world to change around you.

Soli

There have been great advances in understanding the underlying needs that have created this disease of AIDS. There has been a great movement of self-understanding amongst those individuals who are most caught up in it at this time. Those within the gay community who seemingly are most at risk at this time are working very diligently to understand self, to understand society. They are, in many ways, spearheading a new movement that will spread to the rest of the society.

Now, I understand that at this time there is not much sign of this. It seems to be creating even greater demarcation and less understanding. It seems to be creating greater difficulty, more repression. And this is true. This is how it is at this time. However, the energies are moving, they are shifting. As more and more individuals begin to recognize and take responsibility for themselves and understand how they are creating this disease in their lives, it will break down the social barriers, not only from one society to another, but between the individuals within each of those subcultures. There is a tremendous move now of understanding, of acceptance of one by another and it is starting in one pocket, one subculture. It will spread. In the meantime, it is seemingly increasing the demarcation around that subculture. That will also change.

My friends, you are already spiritual, you are already Spirit, you are already God. You are infinite, immortal, eternal, and Universal. You are seeking to go beyond the limiting beliefs of the subconscious mind to understand the Universality that you already are. You are seeking to remember who you are. It is rather as though you had moved into a foreign country and lost your memory. You are striving to remember who you truly are. As you become more understanding of your beliefs and of your subconscious mind, more of the higher energy, the beauty, and the power of the God force that you are will shine through you and throughout the world. God bless you all!

Kyros

Please remember that upon your planet most entities *are* greatly in need of self-healing, so be gentle with yourself and others. Do not feel that you are alone in the process of self-healing, for there are many human and spiritual entities willing to help you in your progress toward wholeness. Be willing to help others along their paths toward wholeness. As individuals are healed, so also is the planet healed.

Enid

Remember that your body isn't you. It's a *vehicle* for you. It's your own favorite child and you want to treat it that way. And remember to always love yourselves, no matter what the invitation to do otherwise. And keep yourselves going ever strongly forward.

Dong How Li

So, my friends, as we leave you, I hope you will have some idea about the importance of *all* of your being and especially your heart as a place of centering in the process. For what you are trying to heal is not only your hearts and your bodies and your minds, but indeed, your very lives, your relationship to life, and your relationship to others. So, I ask you to sit please, with your eyes closed and your palms up in a receptive mode. Allow any thoughts that you have to just keep moving. I ask the Spirit within each of you, your own Higher Self, your own soul, to fill you with its blessing, with its love and its presence so that you have and carry, in all of your being, a sense of yourself. Also carry with you a sense of your fullness and the health that you deserve and indeed have, if you will just allow yourselves to receive it. So, please, in these next few moments of quiet, just enjoy this fullness and this healing. My blessings to you.

SPIRIT SPEAKS . . .

Channeled publications containing universal wisdom and guidance to enhance the material in this book.

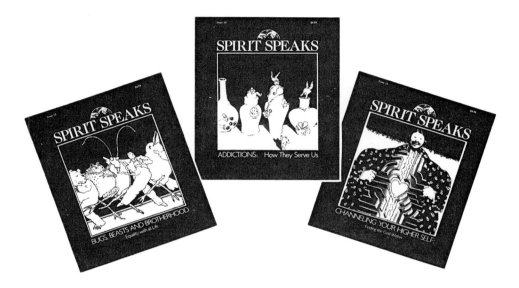

Published every-other-month, every 64-page issue focuses on one specific topic such as love, sex, money, health, addictions, relationships, etc. Each publication contains alternative points of view as expressed by many different Spirit Teachers, including those who have contributed to this book. You will enjoy getting to know them all.

SPIRIT SPEAKS will help you understand more about yourself and how to create a life of joy, excitement, and success. Yes, success! Despite evidence to the contrary, your life is meant to be fun and success-full.

One year subscription to **SPIRIT SPEAKS** (6 issues) is $24. Sample issue is $5.75. To order, or for free information, please write: New Age Publishing Co., P. O. Box 01-1549, Miami, FL 33101. Thank you.